The Cleveland Clinic Guide to

THYROID
DISORDERS

Also in the *Cleveland Clinic Guide* Series

The Cleveland Clinic Guide to Arthritis
The Cleveland Clinic Guide to Heart Attacks
The Cleveland Clinic Guide to Menopause
The Cleveland Clinic Guide to Sleep Disorders

The Cleveland Clinic Guide to
THYROID DISORDERS

Mario Skugor, MD

With
Jesse Bryant Miller

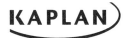

PUBLISHING

New York

© 2009 Kaplan, Inc.

Published by Kaplan Publishing, a division of Kaplan, Inc.
1 Liberty Plaza, 24th Floor
New York, NY 10006

Printed in the United States of America

10 9 8 7 6 5 4 3 2 1

Library of Congress Cataloging-in-Publication Data

Skugor, Mario, 1961–
　　The Cleveland Clinic guide to thyroid disorders / Mario Skugor with Jesse Bryant Wilder.
　　　　p. cm. — (Cleveland Clinic guide series)
　　Includes index.
　　ISBN 978-1-4277-9969-2 (alk. paper)
　　1. Thyroid gland—Diseases—Popular works. I. Wilder, Jesse Bryant. II. Cleveland Clinic Foundation. III. Title. IV. Title: Thyroid disorders.
　　RC655.S679 2009
　　616.4'4—dc22

Kaplan Publishing books are available at special quantity discounts to use for sales promotions, employee premiums, or educational purposes. Please email our Special Sales Department to order or for more information at *kaplanpublishing@kaplan.com,* or write to Kaplan Publishing, 1 Liberty Plaza, 24th Floor, New York, NY 10006.

Contents

Introduction

The Butterfly Under Your Skin

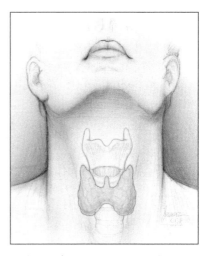

T he butterfly-shaped organ in your throat just beneath the Adam's apple is the thyroid gland. It is small, but it does a lot. The thyroid regulates your metabolism, controls the speed at which many of the factories in your body operate (including the heart), and even helps determine how fast you think. An underactive thyroid (one that doesn't produce enough thyroid hormone) causes everything to slow down, from your heart rate to how fast you metabolize food. This condition, known as hypothyroidism, affects more than ten million Americans. One in ten women over age 30 has an underactive thyroid.

An overactive thyroid revs up the body's factories, causing them to overexert. If untreated, it can lead to weakening of the muscles, thinning of the bone, irregular heart action, and even death.

In this book, I will discuss the various forms of thyroid disease: hypothyroidism, hyperthyroidism, thyroid nodules and goiters, and thyroid cancers. I will introduce you to the most up-to-date treatments, as well as the pluses and minuses of all the available medications. Throughout, case histories culled from my 20 years of treating patients with thyroid conditions will help you understand the array of symptoms and treatment options, as well as recognize when it is time to seek a specialist.

I will also teach you how to detect thyroid nodules—commonly found, usually benign, thyroid tumors (50 to 75 percent of women develop a nodule at some point in their lives)—and will explain the known types of thyroid cancer, most of which are highly curable—especially if caught and treated early. Roughly 5 percent of all nodules are cancerous.

One of the reasons that so many women suffer from thyroid issues is that pregnancy can throw your thyroid out of whack, even if your thyroid was previously healthy. This book will give attention to the particular complications of the thyroid during pregnancy—you will learn what pregnant women need to know about thyroid treatment before and after delivery for their health and for the health of their baby.

Finally, the Internet and magazines regularly tout new thyroid treatments that promise to make you lose weight and become happier and more energetic. I'll discuss these alternative and often controversial therapies, sorting out the well-researched ones from those that need more study, have no basis in research, or are unsafe.

My hope is that reading this book will help you become part of the solution to any thyroid problems you may develop in your life.

Mario Skugor, MD
Staff Physician at the Endocrinology & Metabolism Institute
Associate Professor of Medicine at Cleveland Clinic Lerner
    College of Medicine of Case Western Case Reserve University
    (CCLCM of CWRU)
Codirector of Endocrine and Reproductive Block at CCLCM
    of CWRU

Chapter 1

Your Thyroid

What It Is and What It Does

Thyroid disorders are very common. A 1997 survey estimated that 21.3 million individuals in the United States have some type of thyroid disorder. The number of people who suffer from thyroid problems exceeds the 17.6 million who suffer from asthma or the 15 million who have heart disease.

Almost certainly, goiters—thyroid enlargements caused by iodine deficiency—were common in ancient populations. However, the thyroid gland wasn't identified as an organ until the Renaissance, when studies of the human and animal bodies became more common. Leonardo da Vinci may be the first one who identified the thyroid gland around the year 1500;

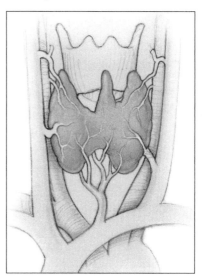

The thyroid is a bow tie–shaped (or butterfly-shaped) gland located exactly where you would wear a bow tie, at the bottom of the neck under the Adam's apple. If you have trouble locating it, tie a necktie tightly around your neck; the thyroid will be the first part of your body to complain. The bow tie's "wings," which are called lobes, are connected by an isthmus—the knot of the bow tie.

however, the first definite description belongs to Vesalius in 1543. The human thyroid was described in early the 1600s. Recognition that goiters are in fact enlarged thyroid glands was documented by Fabricius in 1619. The name *thyroid* comes from the Greek word for *shield* and was coined by Thomas Wharton in 1656.

How Does the Thyroid Work?

The thyroid's job description is to manufacture thyroxine (T4) and triiodothyronine (T3), the two thyroid hormones that control the body's metabolism. Too little thyroid hormone causes hypothyroidism (underactive metabolism). Too much causes hyperthyroidism (overactive metabolism).

Thyroid-stimulating hormone (TSH) is produced in the pituitary gland, the supervisory gland located at the base of the skull, and tells the thyroid how much T4 and T3 the body needs to function normally.

Our bodies use a top-down management system. The hypothalamus portion of the brain (which controls the body's involuntary responses) integrates information from the body, determines how much of the thyroid hormones are needed, and orders the pituitary to manufacture TSH by sending a messenger known as thyrotropin-releasing hormone (TRH) to the gland.

The pituitary passes on the order by sending its messenger, TSH, to the thyroid. The thyroid obeys the order and manufactures more T3 and T4. These newly minted thyroid hormones are then secreted into the bloodstream to relay the pituitary's commands to the cells and organs.

The thyroid hormones are also brought to the hypothalamus and pituitary gland, and there have a regulating effect, inhibiting the production of the TRH and TSH. This completes the regulatory loop.

The thyroid gland stores large amount of thyroid hormones for future use. If the thyroid suddenly stopped making T4 and T3,

Top-Down Management Gets the Job Done

To manufacture much-needed thyroid hormones to control the body's metabolism:

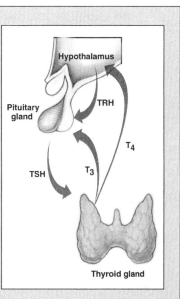

1. The hypothalamus sends TRH to the pituitary.

2. TRH signals the pituitary to manufacture TSH.

3. The pituitary makes the TSH and sends it to the thyroid, to tell it how much T4 and T3 the body needs.

4. The thyroid obeys and manufactures T4 and T3.

5. T4 and T3 swim into the bloodstream to relay the pituitary's commands to the cells and organs.

6. T4 and T3 inhibit production and secretion of TRH in the hypothalamus and TSH in the pituitary gland.

there would be enough hormones to maintain normal metabolism for several months.

What Does the Pituitary Gland Do?

The pituitary gland, which is located at the base of the brain, is the "factory supervisor." It manages not only the thyroid gland but many of the body's other hormone factories, including the adrenal glands at the top of the kidneys, as well as the ovaries and testes. It also secretes growth hormone and prolactin, a hormone primarily associated with lactation.

The pituitary tells the thyroid and other glands when to work harder to produce hormones and decides when to scale back production. When the pituitary decides there is a sufficient amount of thyroid hormone in the blood—which it determines through a kind of feedback loop by sensing the thyroid hormone levels in the blood—it cuts TSH production, and the workers in the thyroid hormone factory (the thyroid cells) go on break.

TSH levels are one way that we can detect thyroid disorders. For example, if a patient's TSH level is high, it indicates that thyroid hormone production is sluggish and that the supervising pituitary has dispatched more TSH than usual to order the thyroid workers to increase production.

What Happens When Thyroid Hormone Production Is Too Slow or Too Fast?

If you think of the body as a machine, thyroid hormones control the rate at which the machine runs. They tell the heart how hard to pump blood, they regulate how fast the intestines move food through, and they determine how much heat our bodies generate.

Hypothyroidism. Too little thyroid hormone causes hypothyroidism. The body lags like an idling engine, which results in:

- Slight weight gain, because energy and fat burn more slowly
- Slower heartbeat
- Chills, since not enough heat is generated
- Slowed muscle reflexes
- Constipation, because the digestive process becomes sluggish

Everything in the body slows down, even thinking and remembering.

Jennifer

Jennifer, a 22-year-old college student, came to visit me because she had a host of complaints.

At her first appointment, she told me that her hair and skin had become coarse and dry despite regular treatment with conditioner and lotion. Her hands ached after taking notes in class or typing a few emails, as if she had carpal tunnel syndrome. She always felt cold, especially her hands and feet. These symptoms were disruptive to her life, but her other symptoms were even worse.

"I constantly feel drained, as if I could doze off at any moment," she said. Yet after sleeping, she never felt rested. Even with nine hours of sleep, she felt like she'd stayed up all night. Similarly, her energy levels prevented her from working out. "After a bike ride the other day, I was shaking and so weak I could barely hold a glass of water! Even standing for a couple of hours makes me feel like I'm going to pass out," she told me.

After surfing the Internet for similar symptoms, Jennifer surmised that she either had an underactive thyroid or was suffering from an adverse reaction to Depo-Provera, the birth control shots she'd begun receiving a couple of months earlier. She called the Cleveland Clinic and made an appointment with me, thinking that an endocrinologist could be the best specialist to sort out her symptoms and find the answer.

"I just want to be a healthy, active 22-year-old woman!" she told me. "Despite doing my best to exercise, I can't seem to lose fat and build muscle. I'm not trying to get skinny, just strong. And I can't focus on things like reading. My eyes get blurry, and I start thinking of something else or just zoning out.

"My memory is going down the drain too. And I'm not as happy as I usually am, and it's driving me nuts."

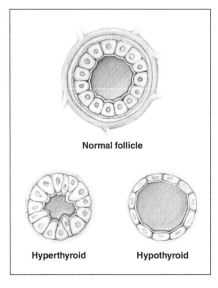

Normal follicle

Hyperthyroid   **Hypothyroid**

I listened sympathetically, knowing from my years of practice how frustrated patients become with these widespread symptoms. I decided to test Jennifer's level of TSH, since it regulates the thyroid gland—one of the body's important hormone factories. The levels are measured by a routine blood test. Blood is taken from the patient's arm and sent to a laboratory for examination.

Jennifer's TSH level was extremely high: over 100 international units per milliliter; the normal range is 0.4 to 5.5. An elevated TSH count is a strong indicator of hypothyroidism. (Sometimes, however, the TSH is just slightly higher than normal, and we may need further tests to confirm whether or not someone truly has hypothyroidism. We will talk more about these tests in chapter 6.)

Hyperthyroidism. If there is too much hormone (hyperthyroidism), the engine races, which causes:

- Weight loss, because the body burns off energy and fat at a more rapid rate than normal
- Fast heartbeat (leading to palpitations)
- Perspiration, from the body overheating like an overworked machine (Hyperthyroid patients tend to perspire even on cool days.)
- Hypersensitive muscular reflexes
- Diarrhea, since food passes through the intestines too quickly

Monica

Monica came to me from Youngstown where she was diagnosed with hyperthyroidism. However, she could not get a timely appointment with an endocrinologist in her area. When she came to my office she was very thin—at least 12 pounds less than her usual weight. She was tired all the time, had a hard time falling asleep, and woke up frequently. She frequently felt hot and had been sweating excessively; she also had a hard time writing because she was experiencing a hand tremor.

Frequently, Monica had been feeling as if her thoughts were racing, and she could not stay focused on tasks. This interfered with her work in a post office. She did not have diarrhea, but her bowel movements were definitely more frequent than before. She was experiencing heart palpitations, especially when undergoing physical activity or when she was under stress. Monica also thought her personality had changed

Signs and Symptoms: What's the Difference?

Doctors often talk about *signs* and *symptoms,* which seem synonymous. But there is a difference:

- Signs are objective facts that a doctor can see. For example, having high blood pressure is considered a sign.
- Symptoms are subjective matters that the patient tells the doctor but that can't necessarily be confirmed. For instance, feeling tired is a symptom but not a sign.
- Sometimes the symptom can also be a sign. An example is a tremor which a patient feels and can also be easily detected by examination.

and that she would explode much more easily than before. This had led to some marital strain too.

"Please, can you help me to feel normal again? This is driving me crazy," she said. Luckily, I could and about two months later she was fine. Her laboratory results indicated she indeed had hyperthyroidism caused by Graves' disease. I prescribed medication that gradually slows down thyroid hormone production, and two months later her thyroid tests had returned to the normal levels. She felt normal and happy again.

The Importance of Iodine

The thyroid needs iodine to form the thyroid hormones T4 and T3. T4 has four iodine atoms and T3 has three. The thyroid extracts the iodine from certain foods we eat—mostly iodized salt and saltwater fish. The iodine is concentrated in the thyroid cells and helps with the assembly of T4 and T3.

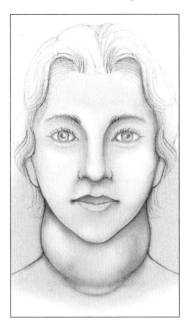

When the thyroid has manufactured and released T4 and T3, the bloodstream ships these hormones to every organ in the body. Each organ has loading docks (or receptors) to receive the hormones inside its cells; thyroid hormones are small molecules and easily enter the cells. When hormones attach to receptors, they signal the cells harboring the receptors to get to work.

What Are Goiters?

A lack of iodine prevents the synthesis of thyroid hormones. The pituitary gland senses the hormone shortage and sends a "rush delivery" of TSH to push for more production. The thyroid struggles to carry out its orders, growing larger under the influence of the high level of TSH.

But without enough iodine, the thyroid still cannot make enough hormones, and eventually the hypothyroid person develops thyroid enlargement, also known as a goiter.

The Iodine-Thyroid Connection

The precise link between too little iodine and thyroid disease has not always been clear. Although ancient Chinese doctors prescribed seaweed to treat goiters, it was not until Bernard Courtois isolated iodine from seaweed in 1811 and Jean-François Coindet of Geneva hypothesized that he could use iodine to treat goiters in 1819, that the wisdom of the ancients was scientifically proved. Even then, some patients were incorrectly dosed and became hyperthyroid, so the treatment was dropped.

Over the next 100 years or so, medical practitioners and healers continued to explore the link between iodine and thyroid disorders. Before the mandatory iodization of salt in the U.S., populations in certain parts of the country—the Midwest, for example—were prone to iodine deficiency. In the early 20th century, it was ten times more likely that a person living in Ohio would have a goiter than someone from Massachusetts, where iodine-rich saltwater seafood was abundant.

Because of the high incidence of goiters in Akron, Ohio, especially among the female population, the Akron public school system and two doctors, David Marine and O. P. Kimball, decided to administer iodized salt supplements to female students. Their experiment worked. As reported in a 1920 journal, *Archives of Internal Medicine,* none of the girls developed goiters. This experiment firmly established the relationship between iodine deficiency and goiter development.

After World War II, the federal government mandated that salt manufacturers iodize their salt to guarantee that all Americans have sufficient iodine in their diets. As a result, goiters are now rare in the U.S. but can be seen in people living in countries where the diet and water lack iodine.

Iodination of the salt led to resolution of the problem of the large number of goiters, and it appears not to lead to development of any adverse health consequences. Hopefully, adequate iodine supplementation will be implemented soon all over the world.

Chapter 2

The Underactive Thyroid

Hypothyroidism

Hypothyroidism (an underactive thyroid gland) is the most common thyroid disorder. The first description of hypothyroidism dates to 1874, when physician Sir William W. Gull described five female patients with profound hypothyroidism, which he called "cretenoid state." He thought this condition was incurable and did not realize that the condition was related to the thyroid. Later, it was noted that the same condition was seen in patients whose thyroid gland was removed surgically, and it was postulated that such a condition was caused by the lack of a thyroid.

In 1890, a report was published regarding a woman with hypothyroidism. She was surgically implanted with a sheep thyroid under the skin, below the breast, and showed immediate improvement in her condition. A year later, in 1891, the first successful treatment using injections of sheep thyroid extract was reported by British physician George R. Murray. In 1892, the first reports appeared of successful treatments using thyroid extracts in oral form.

As we discussed in the previous chapter, the hypothalamus of the brain tells the pituitary gland to produce TSH, which then tells the thyroid how much T4 and T3 the body needs to function normally. But sometimes the thyroid just can't keep up production, and the lack of thyroid hormone begins to affect the body from the top down. Everything from how sharp your thinking is to how much energy you have for daily activities can be affected by under-production of the thyroid hormones, or hypothyroidism.

Recognizing Hypothyroidism

Hypothyroidism is the most common disorder of thyroid function, and it is the state of thyroid gland underactivity. Most of the patients develop hypothyroidism spontaneously, most commonly because of Hashimoto's thyroiditis. However, treatment of some other thyroid disorders leads to permanent hypothyroidism. Patients with thyroid cancers have their thyroid glands removed, leaving them devoid of thyroid hormones. Patients with Graves' disease commonly have their thyroid glands destroyed by radioactive iodine or, rarely, they are removed surgically and the patients are left permanently hypothyroid.

If hypothyroidism is left untreated, it leads to serious suffering and significant functional impairment. These patients feel cold, sleepy, and tired most of the time. They have a hard time remembering, their skin turns dry, their hair may fall out, and constipation sets in. Not fun at all.

The good thing is, adequate treatment leads to complete resolution of the symptoms, and patients can lead an entirely normal life just taking one pill a day.

What Are the Symptoms of Hypothyroidism?

The major signs and symptoms of hypothyroidism include:

- Lack of energy (even after sleeping)
- Feeling cold most of the time and increased sensitivity to cold weather
- Dry, scaly skin; coarse, dry hair; brittle nails; and increased hair loss
- Constipation
- Heavy menstrual periods
- Puffy face
- Hoarse and deeper voice
- Propensity to gain weight
- Muscle aching, stiffness, and tenderness when touched, especially in shoulders and hip areas
- Joint achiness, stiffness, and mild swelling of small joints of the hands and feet
- Muscle weakness, especially in the legs
- Muscle cramps
- Increased cholesterol
- Feeling depressed
- Slowing of the relaxation phase of muscle reflexes
- Elevation of blood pressure, especially diastolic (the lower number in blood pressure readings)
- Difficulties remembering and focusing
- Slowed heart rate (bradycardia)

Severe Hypothyroidism. Severe cases of hypothyroidism often present the following signs and symptoms:

- Lowering of body temperature (hypothermia)
- Slowed speech and movement

Hypothyroidism and Weight Gain

Most people assume that hypothyroidism leads to excessive weight gain, but this actually is not true. The slowing of the metabolism that accompanies hypothyroidism makes it a little easier to gain some weight, but patients who remain physically active despite hypothyroidism gain very little, if any, weight.

However, many patients significantly curtail their activities because they feel tired most of the time. These patients are prone to more weight gain. A small number of patients actually lose their appetite and may lose some weight.

- Jaundice (elevation of levels of bilirubin)
- Tongue enlargement (due to swelling)
- Accumulation of fluid around the heart (pericardial effusion)
- Abdominal distension (due to fluid accumulation called ascites)
- Anemia
- Low blood sodium level (hyponatremia)

How High Does Your TSH Count Have to Be Before Symptoms Present?

The majority of people with mild hypothyroidism—a TSH count between 5 and 15—will not have, or may not notice, any symptoms. With a TSH from 15 to 50, most people will realize they have symptoms, but many will attribute them to other causes, as Jennifer from chapter 1 did. If a person's TSH is 50 or higher, he or she will often recognize that something is wrong and will usually will seek help. It is very rare to find someone who is profoundly hypothyroid, such as someone with a TSH of 200, who is not receiving medical care. But it happens occasionally. Christopher is one such example.

Christopher

Two years ago, a woman brought her 83-year-old father, Christopher, slumped in his wheelchair, into my office. Always on the verge of snoozing, he was unable to manage his own life and seemed oblivious to the world around him.

Another doctor had diagnosed Christopher with Alzheimer's disease and prescribed medication. Most of his family believed he was demented and had decided to commit him to a nursing home.

But his daughter, Julia, challenged the diagnosis, insisting that his current condition resulted from not taking his thyroid medication. His previous doctor had recently retired, and the family had been unable to refill his prescriptions. Within a couple of months, his condition had completely deteriorated.

None of Christopher's other relatives could believe that their failure to regulate his thyroid for a few months could have resulted in such a complete collapse of his ability to function.

After carefully examining my new patient, I interrogated him to determine whether he suffered from dementia or Alzheimer's. "What is your name?" I asked, enunciating each word carefully. The octogenarian wearily lifted his head, leaned forward slightly in his chair, and squinted as if he could barely see me. He exhaled heavily, then rested his head on his hand. After nearly ten seconds, Christopher opened his mouth: "Chris-to-pher," he said, then dropped his head to his chest, as if he were exhausted by the effort.

"Where do you live?" I continued. He opened his eyes again and peered in the direction of my voice. After another ten-second pause, he muttered, "Cleve-land . . . Ohhh . . . hio."

"How many children do you have?" I asked. "What are their names?" Each time, Christopher reflected for seven to ten seconds before formulating a response. All his answers were on target.

I checked his reflexes and, sure enough, his muscle relaxation was very slow. His feet were somewhat swollen, his skin was dry, and his heart rate was 44 beats per minute.

I turned to Julia. "He is definitely not demented. He does not have Alzheimer's," I assured her. "His mind is healthy; it's just very, very slow—like a sputtering engine that's almost out of gas. He must take his thyroid medication. That's the fuel he needs. I guarantee he will improve. Come back and see me in two months."

Extreme hypothyroidism like Christopher's is known as myxedema. If it goes undetected (which is highly unlikely), the patient's metabolism can slow to such an extent that a myxedema coma sets in. In the 19th century, people with a myxedema coma typically sat out of sight in a back room of the family home, quietly vegetating until they died. Their metabolisms simply halted. Although a myxedema coma is extremely rare today, endocrinologists occasionally encounter cases.

Two months later, I walked into my office, and opened the first chart in my computer. I turned to the seated patient, who instantly rose and took my hand between his, shaking it energetically. His daughter stood beside him, beaming. "Thank you! Thank you!" she said.

I looked at the woman, then peered into the man's deeply lined face, trying to remember him. I couldn't place him—until I opened his chart. The change was so dramatic that I hadn't recognized him: Christopher was coherent and active; he was another person. No longer exhausted and slowed by his poor thyroid function, he was articulate, charming, and grateful.

As this case shows, the symptoms of myxedema can be remarkably improved when the disorder is treated. Another important take-home message from this story: it is absolutely essential that patients with severe hypothyroidism stay on their medication.

Detecting Mild Hypothyroidism

Some patients have symptoms even when the thyroid dysfunction appears to be very mild according to test results. This happened to Stephanie.

Stephanie

Stephanie was sleepy throughout much of the day and felt chronically lethargic. She had to push herself to complete tasks, even though she was just 40 years old. She knew that both her mother and sister were hypothyroid, so she suspected she had the condition too. At her request, her family doctor tested her TSH. The result showed she was within the normal range, 3.7, so he declined to treat her for hypothyroidism. In frustration, she sought a second opinion.

After listening to her problems, I had a few questions. Fortunately, first-time Cleveland Clinic appointments are up to 60 minutes long, giving me ample time to really listen. I usually listen to my patients' complaints before asking questions so I can remain impartial; this was my approach with Stephanie.

"Do you or your husband snore?" The frown Stephanie had brought with her to my office deepened.

"Snore? No," she said dismissively. I explained that snoring may indicate that a person isn't sleeping well. This can be due to obstructive sleep apnea, another cause of chronic tiredness. Normally, hypothyroid people don't wake up tired in the

morning. People with obstructive sleep apnea wake up tired. Often, they fall asleep in my office.

I continued asking questions. It turned out that Stephanie often felt cold, even in warm summer weather.

Another question I often ask is whether the patient has gained weight. A weight gain of 20 pounds or more slows you down, so this could be the cause for tiredness rather than the thyroid. Many people immediately assume they have a thyroid condition when they gain weight. Usually, this is not true.

I also asked the patient whether she was on medication because some medications can make you tired. And I asked about sleep and stress. In Stephanie's case, there were no medications and she slept well.

After a careful examination and a discussion of Stephanie's history, I concluded that her symptoms could be related to thyroid abnormality. So I ordered some tests. I repeated the TSH test to confirm the earlier results. The new results—3.5—were essentially the same as her earlier score of 3.7.

Next, I assessed what is called her free T4 level. This measures the amount of T4 traveling freely in the bloodstream as opposed to traveling while bound to proteins. Too little free T4 is a strong indicator of hypothyroidism, even when the TSH is normal.

I also tested Stephanie for antithyroid microsomal antibodies. Microsomal antibodies are produced by the immune system and directed against components of the thyroid cells. These antibodies police the bloodstream and can be measured with a simple blood test. Their presence signifies ongoing thyroid damage that may lead to hypothyroidism (see the section on Hashimoto's thyroiditis on page 22).

Stephanie had two apparently normal TSH tests, with results of 3.7 and 3.5. Her free T4 level was 0.9, which is within the accepted range of 0.7 to 1.8, but her antithyroid microsomal antibody level was elevated at 312; normal is below 10. I thought Stephanie may have mild hypothyroidism and began planning her treatment.

• • • *Fast Fact* • • •

Primary care doctors rarely test for antithyroid
microsomal antibodies when the TSH is normal,
but TSH levels are not the be all and end all of tests.
In my practice, I feel there are times when
additional tests are called for.

• • •

How Could a Normal TSH Level Occur in a Hypothyroid Patient?

Many patients ask me this when their TSH seems normal, but they are having hypothyroid symptoms. In fact, I see quite a few people with TSH levels around 5.0 or 5.5 whose doctors will not treat them because their results are within normal parameters, so they come to me for a second opinion. In my experience, only 5 to 10 percent of such patients will, upon further testing, be found to have hypothyroidism, but it is worth checking out.

One reason that a TSH may be "normal," even though the person is hypothyroid, has to do with the difficulty in declaring a normal range that definitively fits every person in the country. Let's take Stephanie, for example: We know only that her TSH level was 3.5 at the time of testing, not what it was when she was younger. Perhaps at age 20, it was 1. In that case, 3.7 would be high for her and a probable sign of hypothyroidism.

This situation shows why a doctor should never make a diagnosis based on just one number. It is important to treat individual people, not ranges!

How Do Doctors Determine the Best Treatment for Hypothyroidism?

Because everything pointed to hypothyroidism, I prescribed 75 micrograms of an artificial thyroid hormone, Synthroid (levothyroxine), for Stephanie and asked her to see me in two months. The metabolism needs only three to four weeks to readjust after treatment begins, but for thyroid tests to stabilize at new levels, it usually takes six to eight weeks.

Synthroid and all other preparations of T4 (but not T3 and combination T4 and T3) are taken once a day. It is important not to take thyroid hormone supplementation in conjunction with calcium, iron, magnesium, or multiple vitamins that contain these minerals. All of these minerals can impair absorption of the thyroid medication and should be taken three to four hours before or after Synthroid and other preparations of T4.

When Stephanie returned in two months, I immediately noticed that she was more contented. On the first visit, her brow had been furrowed with concern the whole time.

"I have more energy," she said brightly. "I feel happier. But I'm still not 100 percent. A couple of years ago I had even more pep." She asked if turning up the dosage could help. I thought it might, but first I repeated her tests.

Stephanie's TSH had dropped to 1.62, well within normal. Her free T4 was 1.3, also within the normal range. Most primary care doctors would not treat her for a thyroid condition to begin with, let alone increase her prescription. As the initial dosage often needs tweaking, I increased it to 100 micrograms but cautioned her, "If you experience heart palpitations, anxiety, heat intolerance, diarrhea, or insomnia, call me right away." These could be signs that the dosage was too high.

Two months later, Stephanie returned more buoyant than before. "I feel like I'm 20 again!" she effused.

"Do you have palpitations, excessive sweating, shaky hands?" I asked.

"No," she beamed. "I'm fine."

"Just to be sure, let's run the tests again."

Her TSH had fallen to 0.637, and her free T4 had climbed to 1.8. Her levels were still within the normal range, and she said she was at the top of her game. This was the optimum dosage for her particular case. I concluded that she had incipient hypothyroidism.

Who Should Be Screened for Hypothyroidism?

Ideally, everyone over 35 should take a test for hypothyroidism, though such broad testing may not be cost-effective. Nevertheless, this would give doctors a TSH history to compare to later test results. The normal range could then be individualized for each patient.

It's is worthwhile to be screened if you:

- Have a family history of thyroid disease
- Have diabetes or rheumatoid arthritis, which puts you at high risk. You should get tested once a year. About 10 percent of people with diabetes become hypothyroid.
- Have adrenal deficiency or any other autoimmune disease. I recommend an annual test.
- Are over age 60. As we age, we may develop hypothyroidism. Again, an annual test is best.

Causes of Hypothyroidism

As noted previously, hypothyroidism is the most common thyroid disorder, and in the majority of patients, it is caused by Hashimoto's thyroiditis, named after the Japanese physician who discovered it in 1912. (The condition is also known as chronic lymphocytic thyroiditis.)

• • • *Fast Fact* • • •

About one out of ten women over age 30 is affected by Hashimoto's thyroiditis, and the disease is ten times more prevalent among women than men.

• • •

Up to ten million people in the United States have Hashimoto's thyroiditis. Yet roughly two million of them don't know it, largely because they have no symptoms or the symptoms are attributed to a host of other conditions, including aging, stressful lifestyles, lack of sleep, and even Depo-Provera use.

The suffix *itis* in Hashimoto's thyroiditis means inflammation. The thyroid becomes inflamed by attacks from the patient's own immune system, and its tissue is slowly destroyed, eventually resulting in hypothyroidism.

Normally, the immune system (our body's defense system) attacks intruders like viruses and bacteria that would otherwise harm us. When the immune system detects these invaders, it builds and deploys an army of antibodies and lymphocytes (immune cells) specifically aimed at the intruders. They are not supposed to attack the "good guys," the healthy tissue in our bodies. When the immune system does attack healthy tissue—like soldiers firing on their own troops—the condition is called an autoimmune disorder (*auto* means "self"; the body makes war on itself).

Doctors don't fully understand why the immune system attacks healthy tissue. But we do know what happens in Hashimoto's thyroiditis once the invasion begins: large numbers of lymphocytes march into the thyroid gland, massacre thyroid cells, and destroy supporting structures such as connective tissue and blood vessels. Eventually, the thyroid's ability to produce hormones is inhibited. How can a factory make its product at full throttle when it's under attack?

When a thyroid gland that has been invaded by lymphocytes is examined under a microscope, the physician will see both the thyroid structures, which are still recognizable (like a partially bombed-out city), and a large army of lymphocytes spread throughout the tissue. This feature makes it clear where the condition's alternate name—chronic lymphocytic thyroiditis—comes from.

People with other forms of autoimmune disease are susceptible to Hashimoto's thyroiditis. Once the immune system gets accustomed to "friendly fire" (attacking its own troops), there's no telling where it might strike next.

If you have an autoimmune disorder, get yourself checked periodically for Hashimoto's thyroiditis. Some common autoimmune disorders include the following:

- **Rheumatoid arthritis.** The immune system attacks components of the joints.
- **Type 1 diabetes.** The immune cells bombard the pancreas, which is our body's insulin factory.
- **Addison's disease.** The immune cells assault the outer wall of the adrenal gland; John F. Kennedy had this disease.
- **Vitiligo.** A condition suffered by Michael Jackson, in which the immune system attacks the skin pigment cells, leaving white splotches where the pigment-producing melanocytes have been wiped out.

What Are Some Other Causes of Hypothyroidism?

Hashimoto's disease is the most common cause of hypothyroidism, but it is not the only one. Other possible causes of hypothyroidism are as follows.

The Thyroid Itself Is Malfunctioning or Absent. This may be caused by:

- Surgical removal of the thyroid (Development of hypothyroidism is expected after medical or surgical destruction of the thyroid, and a program of thyroid hormone replacement should be launched before symptoms of hypothyroidism set in.)
- Destruction of the thyroid by radioactive iodine
- Congenital thyroid agenesis (the failure to develop a thyroid gland)
- Iodine deficiency or excess

Medications. Certain drugs can also trigger hypothyroidism. If you are taking any of the following, be sure your doctor tests you periodically.

Antithyroid medications, such as methimazole and PTU, are prescribed to treat overactive thyroids. If you take such medicines in high doses or for a prolonged period, hypothyroidism will eventually develop. Careful monitoring is essential.

Lithium is used to treat depression and bipolar disorder. Unfortunately, it also inhibits production and secretion of thyroid hormones. Twenty to 30 percent of people taking lithium develop hypothyroidism, which is usually mild. Patients on lithium who develop hypothyroidism should be treated with thyroid hormone replacement just like other hypothyroid patients. If lithium therapy is stopped, the thyroid gland should be reevaluated two to three months later to see whether it has resumed normal activity. Up to 50 percent of patients who take lithium will develop some enlargement of the thyroid (goiter) under the influence of elevated TSH.

Amiodarone is used to treat heart rhythm disorders (cardiac arrhythmias). It has a high iodine content and interacts with the thyroid gland in complex ways. It can cause hypothyroidism or hyperthyroidism. About 20 percent of patients will experience an increase in TSH for a few months after starting to take amiodarone. It is difficult to decide when and in whom to start thyroid hormone replacement. To complicate matters, these patients' already irregular heartbeats can be aggravated by even slight thyroid overtreatment. Therefore, doctors should closely monitor such patients for hypothyroid symptoms, measuring TSH levels frequently. Hypothyroidism can occur within two weeks after starting amiodarone therapy or as much as several years later.

Interferon-alpha is used to treat patients with hepatitis B and C as well as patients with certain types of malignant tumors, such as kidney cancer and melanoma. About 1 to 5 percent of these patients develop some type of thyroid disorder (thyroiditis, Graves' disease, or hypothyroidism). These conditions usually develop after three months of treatment but can arise at any time during interferon-alpha therapy. Patients who have preexisting thyroid antibodies are at higher risk for development of thyroid problems while on interferon-alpha.

Interleukin-2 (IL-2) is sometimes prescribed for metastatic cancers and leukemias. About 2 percent of patients on interleukin-2 develop thyroid abnormalities, including hypothyroidism.

Perchlorate, which is used rarely and only for diagnostic purposes, inhibits thyroid hormone production and secretion and triggers hypothyroidism. Perchlorate is used as a component of rocket fuel and has been found in tap water in amounts that are considered unsafe. The government is against the regulation of the use of perchlorate, and scientists think that millions of Americans may be exposed to it because of unregulated disposal at rocket launch sites.

Finally, in recent years many new medications have been developed in an attempt to treat different malignancies. Some of these are associated with development of thyroid disorders. Some examples are a drug called sunitinib (Sutent), which causes hypothyroidism evident in biochemical laboratory results in about 85 percent of patients, and sorafenib (Nexavar), which cause hypothyroidism in about 40 percent of patients. The exact significance of these medications for thyroid function is not yet fully known.

Abnormal Materials Invading the Thyroid. Abnormal material can infiltrate the thyroid and replace normal thyroid tissue, inflicting permanent damage. This occurs in sarcoidosis, an autoimmune disorder in which masses of chronically inflamed tissue (granulomas) are formed in various parts of the body. We do not know what triggers this inflammation, but when the invading granulomas replace most of the thyroid tissue, hormone production drops significantly, and hypothyroidism sets in.

Hemochromatosis is a similar condition. In patients with this disease, too much iron is absorbed from the blood and then deposited in other organs, including the thyroid, causing malfunctioning.

Fibrous thyroiditis (also called Riedel's thyroiditis) is an inflammatory thyroid disorder of unknown cause that affects neighboring organs and tissue, such as the parathyroid glands (glands that regulate blood levels of calcium), the vocal nerves just behind the thyroid, the trachea (windpipe), and the chest wall. Inflammation eventually causes the normal tissue to be replaced by dense, fibrous tissue, inducing hypothyroidism and causing the formation of a hard lump in the thyroid area. These patients tend to develop similar inflammations in other parts of the body.

Pituitary Disorders. Pituitary disorders can also cause hypothyroidism, but this is rare. If the pituitary gland doesn't produce TSH, the thyroid gland quits working, and you develop hypothyroidism.

Pituitary dysfunction is usually caused by surgery or pituitary radiation for tumors. Sometimes the tumor itself (either of the pituitary or of nearby structures) causes enough damage to the pituitary gland to trigger hypothyroidism.

An autoimmune disease called autoimmune lymphocytic hypophysitis can also inflame the pituitary. When this occurs, the pituitary cannot produce TSH, and hypothyroidism ensues.

In addition, systemic infiltrative diseases such as sarcoidosis and hemochromatosis can replace normal pituitary tissue, causing a TSH deficiency.

Resistance to Thyroid Hormones. Hypothyroidism may also occur when the thyroid hormone receptors in the cells of the body fail to respond to the free T3 in the bloodstream. This is an extremely rare condition.

Patients with this disorder still produce normal or even increased amounts of thyroid hormones, but their bodies cannot use them; their cells are insensitive to the hormone. These patients are hypothyroid despite high blood levels of thyroid hormones and a high TSH.

Genetic Defects. Other causes can include, very rarely, defects in genes that regulate:

- TSH production in the pituitary (leading to TSH deficiency)
- The TSH receptors in the thyroid cells (leading to insensitivity of the thyroid to TSH)
- TRH in the hypothalamus. If TRH secretion malfunctions, this translates into a TSH deficiency, and the thyroid will not be stimulated to produce thyroid hormones.

Is Hypothyroidism a Permanent Condition?

Hypothyroidism is not always permanent. There are several short-term thyroid inflammations that eventually resolve, enabling the thyroid gland to resume normal activity.

Causes of transient hypothyroidism include:

- Subacute lymphocytic thyroiditis (painless thyroiditis)
- Subacute granulomatous thyroiditis
- Postpartum thyroiditis

These inflammations usually last from several weeks to a few months. At first, you may have temporary elevation of thyroid hormone levels in the bloodstream (from the uncontrolled release of reserve hormone stored in the thyroid gland), but this is usually so mild that it goes unnoticed. After this phase, a brief period of hypothyroidism ensues, followed by complete recovery.

Patients with symptoms and signs of thyroiditis after pregnancy, who have not been diagnosed with Hashimoto's thyroiditis, should be checked three to six months after delivery to see whether their condition has normalized.

Treating Hypothyroidism

In the following chapter, we will discuss some of the ways that doctors treat hypothyroidism. Remember: hypothyroidism is very common, particularly among women who are pregnant or who have given birth. While the effects of the disorder can be very serious—especially when neglected—it is also a very treatable condition.

If you have hypothyroidism, try not to panic or get too depressed. With proper treatment, you can live a perfectly normal life and be symptom-free.

Chapter 3

Treating Hypothyroidism

Before jumping into an explanation of the various treatments, it is important to understand a bit more about the relationship of T4 and T3, the two thyroid hormones that control the body's metabolism.

T3 and T4

T3 is more active than T4 in regulating the body's metabolism; you could say it packs a much stronger biological punch. But the most typical therapy for hypothyroidism is taking T4 hormone.

Why Would I Take T4 if T3 Affects My Metabolism More Powerfully?

The majority of the T3 in our bodies comes from T4 that has converted. When T4 molecules that are cruising the bloodstream encounter cells from the body's organs, they have to surrender one of their four iodine atoms simply to be able to interact with the cells. By surrendering one iodine atom, T4 becomes T3.

Looked at another way, T4 molecules have to lose some "atomic weight" before they can participate in the dance we call metabolism. T4 is too heavy and clumsy to dance with all four of its iodine atoms; it has to shed one and become the more lightweight T3.

Here's where treatment with T4 starts to make sense. By treating hypothyroidism with only T4 supplementation, we allow the body to do some of the work it was meant to do—convert T4 into T3.

Also, prescribing T4 supplements instead of T3 is like fixing a leak in a hose at the source of the leak, where it should be fixed (the thyroid, where there is a shortage of T4 production), rather than correcting the problem at the other end of the hose (or bloodstream) where there is a shortage of T3.

The Principles Behind Hypothyroidism Therapy

Normally, the thyroid releases T4 and T3 into the bloodstream. Most of these hormones quickly attach to proteins circulating in the blood. Only a small proportion of T4 (0.5 percent) and T3 (0.05 percent) circulate on their own, unattached. This is called the free hormone fraction.

The free T3 hormones trigger all biologic action. The free T4 hormones serve as a reservoir from which free T3 is replenished. As discussed above, when it is time to interact with the body's cells, the T4 surrenders one of its four iodine atoms. When this happens, T4 is converted to T3, and T3 conveys the proper messages to the cells.

When prescribing T4, doctors must provide the right amount to achieve normal levels of T3 in the blood.

So How Do We Treat Hypothyroidism?

There is really only one treatment for an underactive thyroid—hormone replacement therapy. This therapy comes in several forms, but essentially it is always the same: patients compensate for their thyroid's underactivity by ingesting thyroid hormone.

The most common method of treatment is a daily dose of T4. Because the absorption of T4 from the intestines into the bloodstream varies from patient to patient, a doctor must consider individual differences when prescribing T4.

Getting the Dose Just Right. So, how do doctors determine the initial T4 dosage? The normal dose is proportional to the patient's weight. For most patients, this is very close to 1.6 micrograms of T4 per 1 kilogram of weight (1 kilogram = 2.2 pounds).

However, many family doctors exercise caution because they don't want to induce symptoms of hyperthyroidism by overtreating the patient. They prescribe a low dose, say 25 or 50 micrograms of T4 per day, then raise the dosage every two months until the symptoms subside.

In my opinion, this usually isn't the best method. Instead, in young or middle-aged individuals who are basically healthy, I begin with a dosage that is a little below the weight-proportional norm discussed above. Then, I adjust as necessary—usually only once, or rarely twice—before the hormone levels normalize. I still warn patients to watch for symptoms of overtreatment such as feeling hot or shaky or having heart palpitations, but this is usually a safe, effective treatment that brings faster results than starting with just 25 or 50 micrograms.

What if I Am a High-Risk Patient?

Some people are at high risk for complications from overtreatment. This group includes elderly patients with weak hearts and young patients with heart arrhythmias that could be aggravated by too much thyroid hormone. With these patients, I begin with a much lower initial dose of T4 and slowly increase it until their symptoms resolve or some negative effect occurs, which would prompt me to lower the dose.

Of course, I tell patients that, because of their risk factors, it may take several dosage adjustments to achieve optimal control of their condition. Explaining the principles behind the treatment is the most important aspect of my interaction with patients.

What if the Right Dose Is Unavailable?

Sometimes the ideal daily dose for a patient is commercially unavailable. The correct dose may be 160 micrograms per day, but manufacturers make T4 only in 150- and 175-microgram sizes. In such cases, I prescribe different doses on different days to achieve the correct average daily dose over the course of the week. For example, a patient who needs 160 micrograms per day could take a 150-microgram pill on four days of the week and a 175-microgram pill on the other three days of the week. This would result in an average of 161 micrograms per day, which is the desired dose.

Of course, this means writing two prescriptions, and most patients will end up with two payments or co-payments. Physicians do not always consider the patient's pocketbook; therefore, some people may need to remind their doctors of any financial limitations. In such cases, I believe doctors should strive to find an adequate dosage that can be achieved with only one pill size. Some compromise may be necessary.

The Scoop on T4 Supplements

The T4 hormone, which is manufactured in pill form, is synthetic, but it has exactly the same chemical composition as the T4 produced and secreted by the thyroid: two amino acids (tyrosine) and four iodine atoms. Recently, there has been a drive to use so-called

Recommended Drugs for Treating Hypothyroidism

Synthroid
Synthroid is the most commonly prescribed medication for hypothyroidism. It is a reliable product that consistently delivers the same dosage of T4 over a prolonged period.

Levoxyl
Levoxyl is similar to Synthroid but may be slightly better absorbed from the intestines into the bloodstream. However, since T4 is metabolized slowly, improved absorption doesn't make much difference except for patients who have difficulty assimilating Synthroid for various reasons, such as intestinal disease. Otherwise, there is virtually no difference in terms of efficacy.

Generic T4 (Levothyroxine)
The generic T4 is much cheaper than Synthroid or Levoxyl, roughly $5 for 50 pills versus $15 to $20 for the same quantity of Synthroid. However, it is as good as brand-name preparations.

"bioidentical" hormones in the treatment of patients. Some patients insist that I use only bioidentical hormones when I treat their thyroid. The fact is, synthetic thyroid hormones are bioidentical—they are exactly the same as thyroid produced hormones.

Several varieties of synthetic T4 are available. The ones I prescribe most commonly are Synthroid, Levoxyl, and the generic form, levothyroxine.

Dosing

Synthroid and Levoxyl T4 pills are color-coded. The purpose of the color-coding is to designate different dosages and prevent mix-ups at the pharmacy and at home.

The drugs come in doses of 25 to 300 micrograms (25 micrograms = 0.025 milligrams). I prefer measuring doses in micrograms instead of milligrams to avoid the decimal point being put in the wrong place and leading to over- or underdosing.

In the most common dose range, 75 to 150 micrograms, pills are divided into smaller-sized increments to allow for fine-tuning.

Is It Important to Stick with One Brand During Treatment?

Although the differences between the various types of T4 are minor, it is very important to stay with one brand. Switching may alter your TSH level and how you feel. The following T4 brands are approved by the FDA.

FDA-APPROVED T4 PRODUCTS

Name of Product	Manufacturer
Synthroid	Abbott Laboratories
Levoxyl	King Pharmaceuticals Research and Development Inc.
UNITHROID	Jerome Stevens Pharmaceuticals Inc.
Levo-T	MOVA Pharmaceutical Corporation
Levothyroxine Sodium	Mylan Pharmaceuticals Inc.
Novothyrox	Genpharm Inc.

Even though all the drug manufacturers label a particular color of pill as 100 micrograms, the pill from one company may actually deliver significantly less of the hormone than a pill from another company. Therefore, switching from one company to another can change your actual dosage and may cause fluctuations in TSH and a return of symptoms.

Because of this, the American Association of Clinical Endocrinologists, The Endocrine Society, and the American Thyroid Association recommend that patients not change from one brand to another. Consistency is a key to successful treatment.

Although the Food and Drug Administration (FDA) administers tests to ensure the bioequivalency of all the different T4 preparations, most endocrinologists are dissatisfied with its testing methods. The FDA conducts its T4 bioequivalency tests with healthy volunteers who have fully functional thyroids, using one dose of T4 (usually 600 micrograms). The blood levels of the volunteers are monitored 30 and 15 minutes before the test and again at the time of the test. Afterward, their blood levels are tracked for 48 hours. The results are adjusted to reflect the participant's baseline value (obtained before the test).

Using this approach, testing the 100-microgram T4 dose and the 112-microgram T4 dose from the same manufacturer yields results that lead the FDA to declare the two doses to be "bioequivalent," but being bioequivalent does not mean affecting patients identically. In fact, I have frequently switched between these two doses to fine-tune therapy for my patients.

All Drugs Are Not Created Equal

Bioequivalency is defined as "the absence of a significant difference in the rate and extent to which the active ingredient in pharmaceutical equivalents become available at the site of drug action when administered under similar conditions in appropriately designed studies." (Try to say that sentence fast!) Although two forms of T4 may be bioequivalent, they won't necessarily be identical. This is an important reason for staying with just one brand of medication.

The good news is that the FDA changed the tolerance ranges in 2008 and now requires different producers to keep their product strength between 95 and 105 percent of the standard strength. This should lead to improvement in consistency between different preparations in the future.

If you knowingly change brands, your doctor should retest you in about two months and adjust your dose if there is a significant change in the TSH level or if your symptoms recur.

Check with Your Pharmacist. In some states, when you go to refill your prescription, pharmacists can switch brands without your consent—or even your knowledge. Often the pharmacist won't even notify the prescribing physician of the change, except when such notification is mandated by state law.

According to recent studies, in cases when pharmacies switched brands without notifying the patient or physician, about 70 percent of the patients were not retested within 90 days, and roughly 40 percent were not retested within nine months. This means that patients have the responsibility for monitoring their medication refills. Ask your pharmacist specifically if your T4 preparation is from the same manufacturer every time you get a refill. Be vigilant and read your medication labels carefully.

Will I Stay on the Same Dosage Throughout My Treatment?

Many people stay on the same dose for 10 to 20 years, but of course, some people need their dosages modified from time to time. For example, in Hashimoto's thyroiditis, when the TSH level is 15 or under, there is still some functional thyroid present and further decline can be expected. Doctors should monitor and retest these patients every six months so they can adjust their medication accordingly.

Occasionally, some symptoms return between annual thyroid checkups. Therefore, it is important to be able to contact your thyroid doctor at any time to schedule earlier appointments if needed. I encourage patients to call me when they suspect their symptoms have returned, not to wait until they are certain that they have returned. I want to intervene sooner rather than later. Whenever you think something is wrong with your health, call your doctor, even if you are not sure.

How Do I Know if I Am Being Overtreated?

Some patients may develop symptoms of overtreatment even while on a stable dose of T4. All patients should be educated about overtreatment symptoms so they can recognize them early and call for help. Sometimes the need for a dose adjustment can be predicted based on a large weight gain or loss. I prefer to recheck my patients if they have a weight change of 10 percent or more.

Overtreatment can lead to warning signs. If you are mildly overtreated you may have symptoms of:

- Feeling hot or shaky
- Heart palpitations
- Difficulty falling asleep
- Excessive sweating

If you are severely overtreated, there may also be symptoms of:

- Anxiety
- Mood swings
- Hand tremors
- Diarrhea
- Muscle weakness—especially thighs and shoulders
- Weight loss

- Inability to sleep
- Abnormally increased heart rate (palpitations) at rest or with even minimal physical exertion
- Inability to focus
- Forgetfulness

If you have any of these symptoms, call your doctor. You may need a dose adjustment.

Women, Take Note. Pregnant women who are hypothyroid typically need to have their dosage upped once or twice before they give birth. After birth, the dosage usually drops to the mother's pre-pregnancy level.

Also, T4 dosage usually needs to be adjusted when a woman starts or stops using birth control pills, when she begins estrogen replacement therapy, and during perimenopause, when ovarian hormonal secretion decreases.

Is It Possible to Be Allergic to T4 Treatments?

I have never seen an allergic reaction to synthetic T4. However, some patients are allergic to the coloring in the pills or to the binding substance (usually cornstarch). In such cases, you can take 50-microgram colorless pills successfully, or you can change to a brand that does not contain cornstarch.

What if I Forget to Take My Medicine?

Taking pills regularly is not always easy, and many people periodically forget. Quite a few of my patients miss one or two doses a month; some miss one or two pills per week. It is important for your doctor to know if you occasionally forget your medication. Don't be embarrassed to say so, and ask how to make up for any missed doses.

I advise my patients to make up for missed pills the following day. For most people, this doesn't create any problems. In fact, some patients have been successfully treated by ingesting their *entire weekly dose* of T4 once a week. I do not endorse this schedule because it results in roughly 50 percent oscillations in T4 blood levels, but in a pinch, with a doctor's guidance, it can be useful.

Taking your missed dose the following day works because T4 has a long half-life in the bloodstream. That means that once you take it, it sticks around for a while. When someone stops taking T4, it takes about seven days for the T4 level in the blood to drop by half. This is why hypothyroid symptoms do not immediately return if you forget to take a pill one day. On the other side of the coin, when we begin T4 therapy, it takes a couple of weeks before the T4 supply builds to a sufficient level in the blood. Hypothyroid symptoms don't disappear overnight.

This means, theoretically, that patients could ingest T4 every other day without adverse consequences. However, this regime would be harder to stick to than daily dosing.

Is It Safe to Take T4 Supplements while Also Taking Other Drugs?

I advise my patients not to take thyroid supplements with other medications that can impede absorption from the gastrointestinal tract into the bloodstream. The following table lists some of these culprit medications.

DRUGS THAT AFFECT T4 ABSORPTION

Calcium supplements	For osteoporosis (bone thinning) and low calcium
Magnesium supplements	For low magnesium and calcium, or other reasons

Iron supplements	For iron deficiency, anemia, or other reasons
Aluminum hydroxide	For treatment of heartburn, gastritis, and peptic ulcer
Colestid and cholestyramine	For blood lipid (fats) abnormalities
Sucralfate	For duodenal ulcers
Raloxifene	For osteoporosis (Only one case has been described in the medical literature. It is possible this happens more often, though, so it is prudent to take this medication at a separate time than T4.)

If you need to take one or more of these, I advise taking the different pills three to four hours apart. For example, you would take calcium supplements several times per day at equally spaced intervals. In this case, a patient could take T4 in the morning and begin the calcium doses at 11 AM or noon.

You can take thyroid hormone at any time of day. Some people are afraid that a nighttime dose of T4 might interfere with sleeping, but that is not true.

Frequently, I am asked about the warning found on the commonly used decongestants. They say that these medications should not be used if one has thyroid disorder. What is meant is that they should not be used if the patient has concomitant hyperthyroidism. This is because an elevated level of thyroid hormones makes the body more sensitive to components of decongestants that can speed up the heart rate and lead to high heart rate. However, this will not happen in individuals who are adequately treated with thyroid hormones because they will have normal blood levels of thyroid hormones and will otherwise be healthy individuals.

Other Kinds of Medicine for Hypothyroidism

Prior to development of synthetic thyroid hormones, treatment of hypothyroidism was accomplished using the extracts of animal thyroids. These preparations are still available and effective. Synthetic preparations of T3 are also available.

What Is This I Hear About Animal Thyroid Supplements?

Armour Thyroid is another preparation for thyroid hormone supplementation. It is made from desiccated pig thyroid glands and delivers both T4 and T3 to the patient's bloodstream.

Ingesting animal thyroids is not a new therapy. For at least 80 years, animal-derived thyroid hormone was the only treatment option. In the 19th century, if you had hypothyroidism, your only choices were to swallow sheep thyroid extract or fry up sheep thyroids and eat them.

At one time, cattle thyroid glands were used, but this practice was abandoned when the risk of Creutzfeldt-Jakob disease (the human version of mad cow disease) was recognized.

Are These "Natural" Drugs Safer than Synthetic T4?

Occasionally, someone will come in to see me and say, "I want to be off Synthroid. I want Armour Thyroid." When I ask why, a common reason is that they want to take only "natural" hormones.

Armour Thyroid is advertised as an "all-natural thyroid medicine." Although this is technically true, I have reservations.

First of all, not all natural things are good for our health. Rattlesnake venom, for example, is natural, but not good for us. Also, besides thyroid hormone, desiccated pig thyroid contains many other substances that are not naturally present in the human body, and we have no conclusive knowledge about how these substances affect humans.

Synthroid is an artificially synthesized hormone, but it is composed of exactly the same substances as the T4 produced by the human thyroid and contains no other unknown substances.

Eating any animal's thyroid has drawbacks. The hormone levels in Armour Thyroid, for example, may be inconsistent from batch to batch since they depend in part on the amount of hormone in the animals, which naturally varies from pig to pig. Thus, a patient's TSH level may fluctuate with each bottle of medication.

The producers of Armour Thyroid combat this problem by mixing desiccated material from different batches and testing for the relative amounts of T4 and T3 in the raw material and in the finished tablets. The ratio of T4 to T3 in the pills is 4.22 to 1. (See the Ratio Conundrum on page 45.)

The manufacturers claim that this approach avoids the problem of inconsistent levels of hormones in their product, and it is true that their pills are more consistent nowadays than in the past. However, I still see unexplained changes in TSH in patients taking Armour Thyroid. (This is important only in patients who are sensitive to small variations in their dose.)

The dosage is measured in grains. One grain equals 60 milligrams and is equivalent to roughly 100 micrograms of synthetic T4. To make it easy to figure the equivalencies between doses of Armour Thyroid and doses of T4, see the box on page 43. Armour Thyroid tablets may have a strong odor; this is not a sign that the pills are spoiled.

Dosing of Armour Thyroid. When taking Armour Thyroid, it is recommended that patients take the whole daily dose at once. Most patients have good results with this schedule, but some need to take the dose in two halves. This may be because the pills contain T3, which has a much faster metabolism than T4.

Armour Thyroid Pill Equivalencies to T4 Doses

Armour Thyroid Pill	Mg	Approximate T4 Dose Equivalent
¼ grain	15 mg	25 mcg
½ grain	30 mg	50 mcg
1 grain	60 mg	100 mcg
1½ grains	90 mg	150 mcg
2 grains	120 mg	200 mcg
3 grains	180 mg	300 mcg

Because of that, the blood level of T3 drops much faster than that of T4. If it drops too much, patients will notice a difference in how they feel later in the day, which can be corrected by splitting the daily dose.

If you miss a dose, do not attempt to compensate by taking a double dose the next time. This can result in high blood levels of T3 and symptoms of hyperthyroidism.

Taking a pill that includes T3 will begin to improve symptoms faster than taking pills containing only T4. But pills including T3 still require about the same amount of time as T4 pills (several weeks) to achieve the full effects of the therapy.

What Other Animal Thyroid Preparations Are Available?

There are other products on the market besides Armour Thyroid that are made from animal thyroids: Westhroid and Nature-Throid. These are made by the same manufacturer and enjoy a small market share.

Westhroid pills are bound with cornstarch; the company developed Nature-Throid for patients who are allergic to cornstarch. It is bound by microcrystalline cellulose instead of cornstarch and is advertised as hypoallergenic. These products are also measured in grains.

The United States Pharmacopeia, an official public standards–setting authority for all prescription and over-the-counter medicines, regulates the quality of animal-derived thyroid hormone preparations by determining the required iodine content of such medicines. Iodine content is an indirect measure of hormonal activity. According to the regulations, a natural preparation should contain no less than 0.17 percent and no more than 0.23 percent iodine.

My Experience with Animal Thyroid Pills. Animal thyroid preparations are not my first choice of therapy because they allow relatively large fluctuations in TSH levels. Most of the variations are within the normal range, but since some of my patients are sensitive even to small TSH fluctuations, I try to avoid these products.

That said, I do have patients who feel well only while taking Armour Thyroid, in spite of the TSH fluctuations. Other patients feel fine one month and fatigued the next. In such cases, I frequently can't be sure if the patient's symptoms are caused by too much or too little hormone, or by something else.

What Other Medications Are Used to Treat Hypothyroidism?

Thyrolar. Thyrolar (liotrix), which is composed of synthetic thyroid hormones, is another preparation offering a combination of T4 and T3 in the same pill. The manufacturing company recommends keeping the pills refrigerated to ensure stable potency. Thyrolar is also measured in grains and comes in the same strengths as Armour

The Ratio Conundrum

Like Armour Thyroid, Thyrolar and other animal-derived preparations are produced to maintain a T4-to-T3 ratio of about 4 to 1. This is based on the assumption that the human thyroid gland produces and releases into the body four T4 hormones for every one T3 hormone.

However, most data that I am aware of shows that the T4-to-T3 ratio inside the thyroid is 15 to 1. Upon release into the bloodstream, the ratio drops to 10 to 1. That means that some T4 is converted to T3 before release.

There is considerable debate among endocrinologists regarding this ratio, but most agree that it should be between 10:1 and 15:1. The question becomes more complicated when one considers data on the relative concentrations of T4 and T3 in tissue outside the thyroid. It appears that different tissues convert T4 to T3 at different rates; thus the T4-to-T3 ratio varies from tissue to tissue.

While we wait for research to shed more light on these areas, we must treat each patient individually and use the therapy the patient finds most beneficial.

Thyroid. The pills contain cornstarch and coloring substances (for color-coding of the pill sizes).

Cytomel. Cytomel (liothyronine sodium) is a commercial preparation of pure T3. It comes in 5-, 25-, and 50-microgram sizes and, like most other thyroid hormone preparations, contains cornstarch.

The T3 in it is very well absorbed. Studies show that about 95 percent of the hormone reaches the bloodstream within four hours of taking the pill. Because of this, patients experience symptom improvement rapidly. The full effect may be achieved in two to three days. That is the upside of T3 used alone.

The downside is that since T3 metabolizes faster than T4, its effects dissipate more quickly. One dose usually doesn't last a whole day, so a twice-daily dose is frequently needed. Otherwise, symptoms may return.

Another potential advantage of using T3 alone is that, in cases of overdosing, stopping therapy leads to much more rapid recovery than when someone overdoses on T4. Also, I use it when I want fast improvement—for example, when someone is profoundly hypothyroid, or in patients with thyroid cancers at certain stages of treatment. (For more on thyroid cancer, see chapter 8.)

If T3 Alleviates Symptoms Faster than T4, Why Don't Doctors Routinely Use T3 to Treat Hypothyroidism?

There are several reasons we routinely prescribe T4 rather than T3:

Dosing Schedule. When T3 is given once a day, patients frequently experience fluctuations in their symptoms and end up needing two daily doses for adequate control. However, simple dosing regimens are very important. All studies on this subject show that patients follow prescribed regimens much better if dosing is once a day rather than two or three times a day. Twice a day doubles the opportunity to miss a pill.

Missing a Dose. Missing a dose of T3 always leads to a temporary worsening of symptoms, and there is nothing we can do to alleviate this.

Overdosing. More people treated with T3 than with T4 experience a slight overdose with the unpleasant symptoms of hyperthyroidism.

It Works! T4 works well for most patients. They feel normal and have no hypothyroid symptoms.

My Bottom Line

I am willing to try therapies that combine T4 and T3 as long as the TSH remains in the normal range and there are no overtreatment side effects.

I explain this to new patients and clearly indicate that I will not prescribe therapy that may be detrimental to their health. I explain combination therapy (taking both T3 and T4) and the controversy surrounding it in more detail in chapter 10.

Why I Use a Flexible Approach

When patients are treated with thyroid hormone replacement therapy, their TSH tells us whether the current dose is adequate. So a TSH test is an invaluable tool for follow-up. But if a physician aims simply to normalize the TSH level and then considers the job done, problems may arise.

Why? Because we have no idea what a patient's TSH was *before* developing hypothyroidism. Just because a TSH level falls in the general category called normal, that doesn't mean it is optimal for every single patient. This is why I firmly believe that every person has to be treated completely individually. What is normal for one patient is not necessarily normal for the next.

This has led to my practice of adjusting the dose of medicine until a patient feels good, even if this means pushing the TSH level to the low end of the normal range (0.4 to 0.6, for example).

As I said earlier, with proper treatment, patients can live perfectly normal lives and be symptom-free. The key is to be properly treated!

Chapter 4

The Overactive Thyroid

Hyperthyroidism

Hyperthyroidism, also called thyrotoxicosis, is the medical term for an overactive thyroid. Hyperthyroidism is much less common than hypothyroidism, but it is still commonly seen in the endocrinologist's office. I see a new patient with thyroid overactivity at least two or three times a week. Most of these patients have significant symptoms interfering with their life, but some have very few symptoms.

Many patients are anxious and less tolerant—their fuse gets shorter. They have problems staying focused on tasks, and their jobs can suffer. In severe cases, there can even be personality changes. Family members frequently tell me, "He's just not the same person anymore." But the effects of hyperthyroidism are physical too.

Recognizing Hyperthyroidism

In some ways, in contrast to hypothyroidism, hyperthyroidism is easier to detect just by looking at someone. An overactive thyroid puts the body on overdrive, causing brain function and even body temperature to work extra hard, as if you were running at high speed all day and all night long. In addition to goiters (enlargement of the thyroid gland), hyperthyroid patients may exhibit brisk muscle reflexes, a rapid or irregular heartbeat (as well as elevated systolic blood pressure), profuse sweating or consistently moist skin, fine hand tremors, and demonstrable muscle weakness. Patients with hyperthyroidism caused by Graves' disease (see page 55) may also present with a bruit (murmur of pumping blood) through the enlarged thyroid gland.

What Are the Signs and Symptoms of Hyperthyroidism?

The major signs and symptoms of hyperthyroidism are:

- Feelings of anxiety
- Irritability (nervousness)
- Difficulty sleeping (especially falling asleep)
- Heat intolerance
- Increased perspiration
- Heart palpitations
- Fatigue
- Muscle weakness, especially in the upper arms and legs
- Forgetfulness
- Weight loss, despite normal appetite
- More frequent bowel movements (even diarrhea)
- Tremor of hands or fingers (fine and symmetric tremor)
- Lighter and less frequent menstrual periods
- Brittle hair

Goiters. Visible thyroid enlargement is sometimes seen in hyperthyroidism. It occurs in most cases of two particular kinds of hyperthyroidism—Graves' disease and multinodular goiter. But there are differences in the degree of enlargement, and these differences are also signs that help the physician determine the condition of the patient.

Multinodular goiters are usually larger than Graves' goiters. The presence of the nodules makes the thyroid bumpy under the fingertips during the examination. The lumps, which can be as large as small grapes, are generally harder than normal thyroid tissue, and some of the lumps may be harder than others.

Usually the multinodular goiter, which is unattached to the skin or tissue, moves independently of other tissue when the patient swallows. If a physician places a finger on the thyroid while the patient is swallowing, he or she will feel the goiter travel under the finger. However, if the goiter remains stationary—i.e., has attached itself to neighboring tissue—the physician should check for cancer in the goiter.

Hyperthyroidism and Age. Elderly hyperthyroid patients may experience shortness of breath (dyspnea), and some will develop an erratic heartbeat known as atrial fibrillation. Other patients experience an inner trembling. Patients often tell me, "I'm shaking inside. I feel this inner shaking."

Some elderly people have apathetic hyperthyroidism, an atypical form of the disorder that is difficult to detect. Apathetic hyperthyroid patients slow down instead of speeding up, so a diagnosis of hyperthyroidism is usually the last thing anyone suspects. Patients with this condition lose weight because of poor appetite. They also have an increased heart rate, but not to the point where they complain of palpitations. It can be a tricky disorder to diagnose properly. That is why I check TSH in elderly patients even when the symptoms are not typical.

Younger people will usually tolerate hyperthyroidism better than elderly people do, and they require a higher degree of clinical severity before symptoms appear.

Detecting Hyperthyroidism

There are a number of signs physicians look for when detecting hyperthyroidism. Take, for example, the case of James.

James

James's mother grabbed a tissue from the box on my desk and handed it to her son. He wiped his forehead, then sopped up the moisture dripping down his cheeks. Although the room was air-conditioned, James was sweating profusely.

I examined 20-year-old James's neck, looking for a goiter, a nodule (lump), or tenderness. He had a slightly enlarged, soft thyroid. No nodules, as far as I could tell. My hands were wet just from touching his throat. He was sweating all over. I assumed that he had a hyperactive thyroid. But we needed several tests before I could be certain.

James related his other symptoms. "I'm anxious, but I'm not anxious," he said, wincing. "It's hard to explain. I feel like my mind goes in a million directions. I can't focus in class. And at night, it's very hard to fall asleep." These are typical hyperthyroid symptoms. James also had minor palpitations, another indicator. Otherwise, the six-foot-tall, athletic youth appeared healthy.

Then James told me he had gained 15 pounds in the last two months. This threw me for a moment. Hyperthyroid patients usually lose weight because they burn energy faster than people with thyroids that function normally. However, 10 to 20 percent of patients with Graves' disease (the most common form of hyperthyroidism) do gain weight.

Further conversation with James revealed the source of his weight gain. He said he was too tired to work out. "I used to run and lift weights every day," he said. "I love exercising. Now I'm too wiped out to do it." His overactive thyroid and metabolism had exhausted him. Although he had scaled back his physical activity, he hadn't cut back on calories. "I still eat like a horse!" He was consuming more than he could burn off, even with a hyperactive system.

James exhibited many of the most common symptoms of hyperthyroidism, and I was reasonably certain that this was the root of his condition. But thyroid conditions can be tricky, so rather than make an assumption, I proceeded to take a careful medical history.

Four years earlier, when he was 16, James was diagnosed with Graves' disease—the most common cause of hyperthyroidism—by his family doctor. He had had some of the same symptoms that he showed in my office but had not put on weight. The doctor prescribed propylthiouracil (PTU), one of two medications used in the United States to treat hyperthyroidism, and the symptoms disappeared. James continued to take the medication as instructed to keep the symptoms at bay.

Two years later, his family set off on a Caribbean cruise. Unfortunately, when they landed on a small island, they drank contaminated water, and all of them developed hepatitis A, a liver inflammation. When James got back from the cruise, his doctor advised him to stop taking PTU. He thought that the medication could adversely affect the hepatitis since one of its potential side effects is elevation of liver enzymes. After his hepatitis resolved, James's hyperthyroidism did not return.

It is standard procedure to stop treatment with hyperthyroid medications after one or two years to see whether the condition has been controlled. About 40 percent of patients will be free of symptoms for a few years. Unfortunately, the disease usually makes a comeback. Ultimately, at least 80 percent relapse.

Now, with James in his sophomore year in college, the symptoms had returned, accompanied by the surprising weight gain. Both he and his family physician assumed he had developed a new condition because weight gain isn't usually associated with hyperthyroidism.

In addition to James's signature symptoms, his TSH was undetectable—less than 0.005. The TSH is usually very low or undetectable in hyperthyroid patients because the pituitary, sensing the excess of thyroid hormone in the blood, curtails or shuts down production of TSH.

But I never make a diagnosis based on just one number. To be 100 percent certain, I administered two other tests to measure the levels of free T3 and free T4 in James's blood. I expected these tests to confirm his hyperthyroidism, even though he didn't have all the typical symptoms. Few patients do.

Because of James's previous history, along with his slightly enlarged, soft thyroid and lack of nodules, I suspected that Graves' disease was the cause of his hyperthyroidism.

How Do Doctors Determine the Best Treatment for Hyperthyroidism?

Although diagnosing hyperthyroidism is fairly simple (by using blood tests for TSH and thyroid hormone levels), it is also important to find out the cause of the condition. Without knowing the cause, we can't determine the best course of treatment.

See Discovering the Cause of Hyperthyroidism on page 65 for a more detailed explanation of the detection process.

Who Should Be Screened for Hyperthyroidism?

In my opinion, anybody exhibiting symptoms of anxiety, increased heart rate or any heart arrhythmia, unexplained weight loss, significant fatigue, excessive sweating, or intolerance to heat should be checked for hyperthyroidism. Elderly patients who show functional decline and/or have a goiter should be checked too.

Causes of Hyperthyroidism

While the symptoms and signs listed previously in this chapter are common to all types of hyperthyroidism, some symptoms are specific to Graves' disease, also known as diffuse toxic goiter. Graves' disease is the cause of between 70 percent and 80 percent of cases of hyperthyroidism.

With Graves' disease, the thyroid typically doubles in weight from roughly one ounce to two ounces (although it could be smaller) and sometimes to larger than twice its original size. The gland feels smooth to the touch because there are no nodules, and it is usually softer than normal. If a highly hyperthyroid patient has a larger goiter, the physician can hear blood pulsing through the goiter with a stethoscope. This is a telltale sign of Graves' disease.

• • • *Fast Fact* • • •

Women of any age are 10 to 15 times more
likely to contract Graves' than are men.

• • •

What Is Graves' Disease?

Graves' is an autoimmune disorder in which the immune system produces antibodies that are aimed to attack the thyroid gland. The unusual feature of these antibodies is that instead of causing damage to thyroid cells (as we see in Hashimoto's disease—see chapter 2), they attach to the cell's receptors, which normally serve as docking stations for TSH. From there, the antibodies—known as thyroid-stimulating immunoglobulins (TSI)—send a false message, tricking the thyroid into producing hormone against the orders of the pituitary. The thyroid gland becomes an unwitting rebel and manufactures more T3 and T4 than the body needs.

Of course, the vigilant pituitary, sensing the overabundance of hormone in the blood, tries to reassert its authority by halting TSH production. However, the thyroid persists in obeying the misdirection of the thyroid-stimulating immunoglobulins.

Because the pituitary shuts down TSH production, a Graves' patient's TSH level is usually very low or undetectable, so a routine blood test for TSH is an excellent way to screen for the disorder. Also, hyperthyroid patients with Graves' disease usually have an excess of T3 and T4 in their blood.

In children with Graves' disease, the growth process may speed up so that they are larger than their peers.

Graves' Eye Disease. In about 30 percent of people with Graves', the disease sometimes causes eye changes. This condition is called Graves' eye disease (Graves' ophthalmopathy).

The symptoms and signs of Graves' eye disease vary greatly in severity. In the mildest form, patients complain of a gritty feeling in the eyes, like sand. But there are no visible changes.

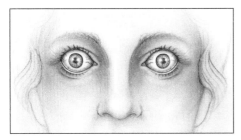

If the condition is moderate, patients will have prominent eyes, like former First Lady Barbara Bush.

Some patients seem to always be staring. When they look down, the whites stand out conspicuously because the upper eyelids tend to stay up or lag, exposing more of the sclera (whites). This symptom is called eyelid lag. However, eyelid lag does not always indicate thyroid eye disease; some people's eyelids lag naturally.

In severe cases, patients develop exophthalmos, a disorder in which the eyeballs bulge from the eye sockets, as if popping out of the head. The condition is caused by an increased amount of fat tissue and muscle swelling behind the eyeballs, pushing the eyes forward in their sockets. The swelling is caused by inflammation triggered by antibodies attacking the tissue behind the eyes. Bulging eyeballs make it difficult for patients to close their eyes. When they sleep, their eyes remain partly open. This causes the corneas to dry out, which can lead to ulcers and loss of vision.

Treatment for milder cases includes artificial teardrops and covering the eyes when sleeping with eye masks, like those provided on airplanes for overnight flights. In addition, protruding eyes may lose ability to move synchronously; therefore, patients may experience double vision (diplopia), which can be corrected with special glasses.

In more severe cases, the blood vessels in the eyes—and sometimes the lids—swell and redden. And, in the most extreme cases, which represent 3 to 4 percent of people with Graves' eye disease, the eye-muscle swelling exerts pressure on the optic nerve and, if left untreated, can cause atrophy of the nerve and blindness.

If you have Graves' eye disease, you need to consult both an endocrinologist and an ophthalmologist with extensive experience in treating thyroid eye disease.

For more serious cases, patients are given steroids. People with the most severe conditions may need eye surgery that will suck up the fat behind the eyes.

For most people, the condition is mild and improves on its own after treatment for hyperthyroidism. But with some patients, the disorder worsens. We don't know why. The only thing we know for certain is that worsening of the disease is associated with smoking. If you smoke and have Graves' eye disease, your condition is more likely to deteriorate.

Studies suggest that Graves' eye disease is more severe in people who have higher levels of thyroid-blocking immunoglobulins, or TBI. These antibodies counter the action of thyroid-stimulating immunoglobulins by blocking the thyroid receptors. Usually, their numbers are smaller than those of thyroid-stimulating immuno-globulins, so the action of the latter typically dominates thyroid function. It is like a football game played with only running backs on one team and blockers on the other. In this game, there are usually many running backs and only a few blockers.

Other Graves'-Specific Symptoms. Another Graves' disease–specific symptom is pretibial myxedema, not to be confused with the hypothyroid condition myxedema. Patients develop patches of thickened, reddened skin on their shins and the back of the feet. This condition is also called Graves' dermopathy.

What Are Some Other Causes of Hyperthyroidism?

Graves' disease doesn't cause all hyperthyroidism—there are other causes.

Toxic Adenomas. Sometimes a thyroid nodule (a lump of thyroid tissue forming a tumor) acquires the ability to produce hormones on its own and does not respond to TSH anymore. Such nodules are called toxic adenomas and act as independent hormone factories, producing T4 or T3 (or both).

With both the toxic nodule and the thyroid manufacturing T4 and T3, the supply of hormone in the bloodstream soon becomes overstocked. In response, the pituitary cuts off TSH production, which signals the thyroid to halt hormone production. The thyroid obeys the pituitary's orders; but the nodule, which is autonomous, more or less shrugs its shoulders and says, "I'm not listening to the central government. I'll make as much hormone as I want." The result is hyperthyroidism.

Some patients with toxic adenomas have full-blown hyperthyroidism, while others have only slight abnormalities on lab tests and few if any symptoms.

A toxic adenoma may appear singly in the gland or as a part of a multinodular goiter. Nodules are discussed in more detail in chapter 7.

Thyroiditis. Inflammation of the thyroid gland (thyroiditis) can also cause hyperthyroidism. When the thyroid becomes inflamed, the thyroid's reserve hormones are dumped into the bloodstream, leading to temporary hyperthyroidism.

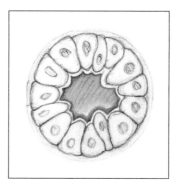

The thyroid gland is composed of follicles that look like small balloons. These balloons are the warehouses where T4 and T3 reserves are stored. There are enough hormones in the follicles to support the body for a couple of months, even if the thyroid shuts down.

Inflammation of the thyroid attacks and ruptures the warehouse walls (the skin of the balloons), and the hormone reserves spill out of the cracks, gushing into the bloodstream and causing

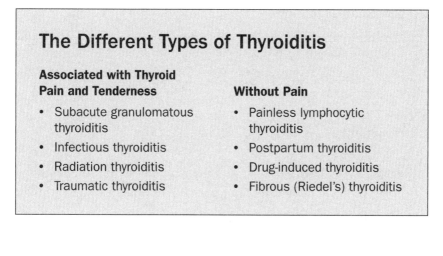

The Different Types of Thyroiditis

Associated with Thyroid Pain and Tenderness

- Subacute granulomatous thyroiditis
- Infectious thyroiditis
- Radiation thyroiditis
- Traumatic thyroiditis

Without Pain

- Painless lymphocytic thyroiditis
- Postpartum thyroiditis
- Drug-induced thyroiditis
- Fibrous (Riedel's) thyroiditis

temporary hyperthyroidism. When the reserve supply is exhausted, the patient may become hypothyroid.

There are several types of thyroiditis, some of which are associated with pain and tenderness; others are painless.

Subacute Granulomatous Thyroiditis. Unlike most forms of thyroid disease, which are more prevalent in women, subacute granulomatous thyroiditis is equally distributed between women and men. This condition has been called many names in medical literature: de Quervain's thyroiditis, subacute thyroiditis, subacute nonsuppurative thyroiditis, and giant cell thyroiditis. It usually occurs after a viral illness, such as a flu or cold—typically, two to eight weeks afterward.

It is not clear whether viral infection spreads to the thyroid gland or simply triggers inflammation without viral invasion of the gland itself. We do know that this is not an autoimmune disorder and that people are genetically predisposed to develop it.

When present, the pain can start suddenly or develop gradually. It may be limited to the thyroid, but often it spreads to the jaw or ears, and it may be misdiagnosed as an ear infection, strep throat, or temporomandibular joint problems (TMJ). Subacute granulomatous thyroiditis is frequently accompanied by fever, muscle aching, and fatigue, which further increase the similarity to an ordinary infection.

A thyroid function blood test will reveal the hyperthyroidism because inflammation damages the thyroid, causing it to release a burst of thyroid hormone into the bloodstream.

Fortunately, painful thyroiditis usually heals by itself in two to six weeks. Over-the-counter painkillers can be used, or sometimes the physician will prescribe steroids.

In about 15 percent of cases, the condition permanently damages the thyroid, which is then unable to produce enough hormones. In such cases, the patient becomes hypothyroid for life and must be treated accordingly.

Once the thyroiditis resolves, it is unlikely to return. Only 1 to 2 percent of patients ever experience another episode.

Infectious Thyroiditis. Infectious thyroiditis (also called acute suppurative thyroiditis) is a very rare form of thyroiditis and is caused by bacterial infection in the thyroid. The infection causes pus to collect, forming an abscess in the thyroid gland. Today, we see such cases in patients with immune-system deficiencies and in children if an infection travels from the voice box area to the thyroid. Treatment involves both antibiotics and surgery to drain the pus.

Radiation Thyroiditis. This form of thyroiditis occurs occasionally in patients who have been treated with radioactive iodine for Graves' disease. These patients develop thyroid pain and tenderness for five to ten days after receiving treatment. There may be some worsening of hyperthyroid symptoms. However, the pain is usually mild and disappears in a few days.

Traumatic Thyroiditis. As its name suggests, this kind of thyroiditis may be triggered by trauma associated with a thyroid biopsy or surgery. It can also be caused by a seat belt constricting the thyroid during a car accident, or by someone squeezing or feeling the gland too vigorously. Both the pain and hyperthyroidism caused by traumatic thyroiditis are short-term.

Painless Lymphocytic Thyroiditis. Painless lymphocytic thyroiditis, also known as subacute lymphocytic thyroiditis or silent thyroiditis, is responsible for up to 10 percent of all cases of hyperthyroidism. Some doctors think it is a variant of Hashimoto's thyroiditis because it has many of the same features: high levels of antimicrosomal and antithyroglobulin antibodies, as well as a tendency to strike where there is a family history of autoimmune thyroid disease.

Thankfully, the hyperthyroidism is only temporary and usually lasts from two to eight weeks, after which the condition completely resolves. In some patients, there is a brief hypothyroid phase after the hyperthyroidism subsides.

Eventually, about half of all patients who have had painless lymphocytic thyroiditis develop permanent hypothyroidism, so having regular checkups is a good idea.

Postpartum Thyroiditis. Postpartum thyroiditis is similar to silent thyroiditis. As the name suggests, it occurs after pregnancy. For details, please see chapter 9.

Drug-Induced Thyroiditis. Drug-induced thyroiditis can occur in patients treated with interferon-alpha, interleukin-2, amiodarone (Cordarone), and lithium. Some patients experience a brief hyperthyroid phase.

Fibrous (Riedel's) Thyroditis. Fibrous thyroiditis is a rare disease. In this disorder, a dense connective tissue (scar-like tissue) replaces the normal thyroid tissue and grows outside the thyroid, invading the surrounding structures such as the wind pipe, esophagus, and muscles. Patients usually develop hypothyroidism, but the most prominent symptom is a hard mass growing in the thyroid bed. The process may lead to difficulties with breathing and swallowing. At this time we do not know the cause of this disorder. Surgery is sometimes necessary to relieve pressure to the trachea and esphagus.

Iodine-Induced Hyperthyroidism. Iodine-induced hyperthyroidism is usually seen in patients who have a multinodular goiter—an enlarged thyroid with multiple nodules. Iodine delivered in the blood to the thyroid may cause a nodule to use the iodine and manufacture an overabundance of thyroid hormones, leading to hyperthyroidism.

This type of hyperthyroidism tends to affect people over 60 because nodules are much more common in this age group. Also, many older people get CT scans with dye made with large amounts of iodine. Another source of extra iodine is the drug amiodarone (Cordarone), prescribed for people with heart rhythm disorders. It is about 37 percent iodine.

Factitious Hyperthyroidism. Factitious hyperthyroidism occurs when the body has too much thyroid hormone taken as thyroid hormone supplement. This can happen accidentally—for example, if a pharmacist or a physician gives out the wrong prescription—or on purpose, such as when someone takes thyroid hormone purposely to lose weight (a very dangerous thing to do—see chapter 10 for more information).

Ingesting thyroid hormones found in some meat products could also cause this kind of hyperthyroidism. In the mid-1980s, a slaughterhouse in Minnesota added an extra ingredient to its ground beef recipe: cow thyroids. The thyroids were harvested, probably inadvertently, during gullet trimming, a process that strips meat for hamburger from the cow's larynx.

After the meat was packaged and sold, an outbreak of hyperthyroidism soon spread through nine adjacent counties in three states: southwestern Minnesota, southeastern South Dakota, and northwestern Iowa. In all, 121 cases were reported.

After that outbreak, the United States Department of Agriculture (USDA) prohibited gullet trimming in all USDA-inspected slaughterhouses.

A similar cluster of cases occurred in Poland from consumption of sausage made with pig thyroids.

In the 1980s, a woman became hyperthyroid from eating beef patties made from a cow her husband slaughtered on their farm. The patties included gullet trimmings. Her husband preferred eating other parts of the animal and never became hyperthyroid.

These types of cases are extremely rare nowadays.

Subclinical Hyperthyroidism. Subclinical hyperthyroidism is a mild version of the condition with no apparent symptoms. It occurs when the TSH is suppressed and the free levels of T4 and T3 remain normal.

A large study of Americans found that about 0.7 percent of individuals have subclinical hyperthyroidism. It is most common in women, African Americans, and elderly patients.

Causes of subclinical hyperthyroidism include:

- Intentional suppression of TSH with thyroid hormone
- Multinodular goiter (especially in the elderly)
- Mild Graves' disease
- Toxic adenoma

The major cause of subclinical hyperthyroidism is overtreating hypothyroid patients by giving them too much thyroid hormone. This is done intentionally when treating patients with thyroid carcinomas because it helps keep the cancer from recurring.

The potential risks of having untreated subclinical hyperthyroidism are the development of osteoporosis and adverse effects on heart function (atrial fibrillation is more common in these patients than in the general population).

Such problems have occurred in people whose TSH was not only lower than normal, but lower than 0.1 microunits per milliliter.

Are There Any Rare Causes of Hyperthyroidism?

Though hyperthyroidism is typically caused by the conditions or illnesses previously described, there are cases in which a patient's overactive thyroid has been triggered by something more rare.

Struma Ovarii. In struma ovarii, renegade thyroid tissue grows inside the ovary.

When a lump of thyroid tissue appears out of its normal location, it is called an ectopic thyroid. In Latin, *ec* or *ex* means "out of" and *topos* means "place." (An ectopic pregnancy is an out-of-place pregnancy—one that is implanted outside the uterus, usually in the fallopian tubes.)

An ectopic thyroid can become autonomous and produce thyroid hormone, causing hyperthyroidism. It does not respond to orders from the pituitary. A man may develop an ectopic thyroid in his testicles, though this is extremely rare.

Cancer Metastasis. The widespread metastasis of thyroid cancer may cause hyperthyroidism because cancerous thyroid tissue can manufacture T4 and T3. Cancerous tissue is a poor maker of thyroid hormone, and it takes large amount of tissue to cause hyperthyroidism.

Discovering the Cause of Hyperthyroidism

As mentioned earlier in this chapter, it is relatively easy to successfully diagnose hyperthyroidism using blood tests and by checking hormone levels. But without knowing the root cause, the thing that is pushing the thyroid into overdrive, we can't properly determine an effective course of treatment.

What Tests Are Used to Determine the Underlying Cause of Hyperthyroidism?

Radioactive Iodine Uptake and Scan. A radioactive iodine uptake and scan is usually the best test to distinguish among common causes: Graves' disease, toxic nodule, thyroiditis, and factitious hyperthyroidism. For this test, the patient swallows a pill containing a very small, safe amount of radioactive iodine. The patient's thyroid is later scanned by a special gamma-ray camera to obtain a picture of the gland. (For more information on the scan, see chapter 6.)

Because the thyroid naturally extracts most of the iodine in the blood as raw material for building thyroid hormone, the thyroid will absorb a significant amount of the radioactive iodine if it is actively producing hormone.

In Graves' disease, the uptake is high, and the radioactive iodine is evenly distributed throughout the thyroid gland. In cases of toxic nodule, there is an intense uptake in the tumor itself but very little uptake in the rest of the thyroid. If a patient has thyroiditis or has taken too much thyroid hormone, the uptake will be very low, and the thyroid gland will be barely, if at all, visible on the scan.

Sometimes the radioactive iodine test cannot be used. Radioactive iodine must not be given to a pregnant woman because it could endanger the fetus. Also, when a patient's body is loaded with nonradioactive iodine, the scan won't work.

In such cases, we must rely on blood tests, observation, and sometimes ultrasound exams to determine the exact cause of the hyperthyroidism.

Measuring Thyroglobulin. Patients who secretly take thyroid hormones are rare but present certain unique problems. The few times I have encountered such patients, it has been difficult to get them to admit that they are taking the hormones.

Few of my patients appear to derive benefit from being ill. Their family members expend a great deal of time and energy attempting to help them find a reason for their ailment and to help them feel better. Why would someone take thyroid hormone and made herself sick? One patient did it in attempt to control her weight and has persisted despite all the unpleasant symptoms of hyperthyroidism.

When, after obtaining the radioactive iodine scan and uptake measurement, I suspect a patient is ingesting thyroid hormone on the sly, I measure the thyroglobulin level in the blood. In cases of thyroiditis, the thyroglobulin will be elevated, sometimes very high, but with factitious hyperthyroidism, it is very low, usually below the level of detection. This is a tip-off that someone is secretly taking thyroid hormone.

The most useful test for ruling out Graves' disease in patients who do not admit to ingesting hormone is the thyroid receptor antibodies (TRAbs) test, a simple blood test. If the test detects thyroid receptor antibodies (thyroid-stimulating immunoglobulins and thyroid-blocking immunoglobulins), the patient has Graves' disease. If the thyroid receptor antibodies test is negative, we know the patient doesn't have Graves' disease.

Ultrasound. Ultrasound examination is rarely used in evaluating hyperthyroidism, but it can be useful especially in hyperthyroid patients who are taking amiodarone. There are two different ways this drug can produce hyperthyroidism, and I try to determine whether the patient is suffering from drug-induced thyroiditis or iodine-induced hyperthyroidism (from the large amount of iodine in amiodarone).

An ultrasound image may help solve this problem. When I look at an ultrasound of the thyroid, there will be no significant blood flow through the gland if the patient has amiodarone-induced thyroiditis. On the other hand, if the patient has iodine-induced hyperthyroidism, the image will show increased blood flow.

In this chapter, I described a variety of disorders that can cause hyperthyroidism. But in the usual practice, the vast majority of the cases will be caused by Graves' disease, toxic adenoma, or subacute thyroiditis. Distinguishing between these is not hard in most cases and treatments are available for each case. I will address these treatments in next chapter.

Chapter 5

Treating Hyperthyroidism

T here are several definitive treatment options for hyperthyroidism, and the choice depends on:

- The severity of the symptoms. If the symptoms are severe, your doctor may try to alleviate some of them even before figuring out the underlying cause.
- The cause of the condition. Treatment for Graves' disease can be different from the treatment for hyperthyroidism caused by a tumor or a multinodular goiter.
- The patient's preferences

Treating Severe Symptoms

Some patients' symptoms are so severe that they need immediate treatment. For example, if an elderly patient's heart rate is dangerously fast because of hyperthyroidism, he or she may be at risk for heart failure or a heart attack. Slowing the heart rate is a priority. Shaking is another symptom I would treat first if it is severe enough to impair the patient's ability to function.

In such cases, I use a special class of medications, beta-blockers, to slow the heart rate and relieve some of the patient's anxiety, allowing for better sleep. Patients generally feel better quickly with this approach. Then I determine the cause of the condition and decide on a long-term therapy.

There are many medications in the beta-blocker group. The two that endocrinologists use most often are atenolol (Tenormin) and metoprolol (Lopressor, Toprol XL). But beta-blockers are not for everyone; they can aggravate asthma and make it harder to control blood sugar in people with diabetes.

I may sometimes prescribe antithyroid medication to stop the thyroid from producing T4 and T3. This helps when the cause is Graves' disease or a tumor that autonomously produces hormones, but not if the patient has thyroiditis (because the thyroid is already shut off).

Treating Thyroiditis

If the cause of the overactive thyroid is thyroiditis, there is usually no need for any thyroid-specific treatment (although your doctor may recommend treating some of the symptoms for immediate relief). Eventually, the body heals itself of thyroiditis. Nevertheless, the patient must be monitored after the inflammation subsides because hypothyroidism may develop later.

Treating Hyperthyroidism with Medication

The association of an enlarged thyroid and symptoms of hyperthyroidism was recognized in the beginning of the 18th century. In 1830, Irish physician Robert James Graves discovered that several of his patients who had an enlarged thyroid gland also suffered a rapid or irregular heartbeat and enlarged and protruding eyes. Graves postulated that a disorder of the thyroid gland was the cause of these conditions, and he documented that women were suffering from this condition much more frequently than men. His theory was confirmed by the German physician Karl Adolph Von Basedow. Basedow also realized that this condition caused weight loss and nervousness. He proposed that excessive iodine could be a contributing factor to the illness. However, there were no appropriate medical treatments for a long time. The first drug approved for use in treatment in the U.S. was propylthiouracil (PTU) in 1947.

What Medications Are Used to Treat Hyperthyroidism?

There are two medications used to treat hyperthyroidism in the U.S.: propylthiouracil and methimazole (Tapazole). European physicians also prescribe carbimazole, which turns into methimazole upon absorption into the body.

The drugs are similar. Propylthiouracil and methimazole consistently bring hyperthyroidism under control, usually within several weeks. If symptoms persist, it is usually because the patient isn't taking the medicine regularly.

Both drugs halt the production of thyroid hormone. One advantage to using PTU is that it also prevents conversion of T4 into T3. Another big advantage of PTU is that it can be taken during pregnancy. In fact, it is the only treatment other than surgery that can be used for pregnant women.

A disadvantage of PTU is that it is manufactured only in 50-milligram units and has to be taken three times per day. The daily dose can vary from 50 to 900 milligrams, depending on the severity of the condition, so a patient may have to take up to 18 pills a day!

An advantage of Tapazole is that it can be taken once, twice, or three times a day, not just three times as with PTU. The maximum dose is 60 milligrams per day. Pills come in sizes of 5 or 10 milligrams.

I prefer Tapazole because I can frequently prescribe it in one daily dose, which makes it much easier for patients to stick to their medication routine. In addition, studies suggest that methimazole controls symptoms a little faster than PTU. I usually start by prescribing Tapazole in 20-milligram dosages twice a day, or a 30-milligram dose once a day in milder cases. After five to seven weeks, I lower the dosage to 10 or 20 milligrams once a day. Once the thyroid hormone production is normalized, even a 5-milligram dose once a day may be enough to keep it normal.

Are There Any Side Effects to These Medications?

Methimazole and PTU cause side effects in 1 to 3 percent of patients. The most common are skin rash, itching, hives, abnormal hair loss, and skin pigmentation problems. Less common side effects include swelling, nausea, vomiting, heartburn, loss of taste, joint or muscle aches, numbness, and headache. Both drugs can also cause liver damage, and although it happens rarely, severe liver damage and even death may result. It is very important when taking these medications to remain in contact with your prescribing physician and to have regular follow-up visits or check-in calls so your doctor can monitor your progress and make sure the more serious side effects do not harm you.

Unfortunately, both medications have another severe side effect called agranulocytosis, which is extremely rare but can be fatal. To ease your anxiety, let me put how rare it is into perspective for you:

Red Flag

When taking medication for hyperthyroidism, any infection—from a sore throat to a boil—should put you on red alert.

in the United Kingdom, over a 40 year period with tens of millions of prescriptions of both medications, 115 cases of agranulocytosis were reported, with six fatalities. Nevertheless, the disease may strike any hyperthyroid patient on PTU or Tapazole at any time.

Agranulocytosis is an idiosyncratic reaction with no known trigger. It is extremely dangerous because it strikes without warning and can annihilate most of the body's immune system by attacking immune cells called granulocytes.

Granulocytes are the body's standing army, protecting it from invading bacteria. They make up 70 percent of the body's white blood cells. If the granulocyte army were suddenly wiped out, bacteria would invade and overwhelm the body with acute infections.

Because agranulocytosis is so deadly, attacking suddenly and surreptitiously, hyperthyroid patients must be constantly on guard.

Agranulocytosis occurs twice as often with PTU as with Tapazole. With PTU, there is no relation between dose and risk; the risk

Emergency Plan for Agranulocytosis

If you have any sign of an infection, go to an ER immediately. *Don't go to bed and visit your doctor the next day. Head immediately to the ER.* You don't know whether you have an ordinary infection or agranulocytosis, and you must find out immediately.

Take your medicines with you to the ER. Show them to the staff, and explain your symptoms. They will immediately test your white blood count. If it is elevated, this shows that you have an ordinary infection.

But if the white blood count has dropped significantly, it is likely that agranulocytosis has developed. You will be hospitalized and taken off thyroid medication immediately, and a culture will be taken to find out what microorganism caused the infection. Intravenous antibiotics will be administered to fight off bacteria until the white blood cells recover.

is always the same. But when a patient is pregnant or breast-feeding, PTU is the only option.

With Tapazole, the risk of developing agranulocytosis is related to dosage; the lower the dose, the lower the risk.

I never recommend PTU or Tapazole as a permanent treatment for hyperthyroidism unless the patient absolutely insists. A more effective approach is radioactive iodine ablation, which is described below. This treatment avoids the likelihood of agranulocytosis and the necessity of rushing to the ER every time you have a simple infection, such as a cold or a urinary tract infection.

Patients have asked why I don't monitor them for agranulocytosis. Quite simply, there is no way to do so successfully. Checking the white blood count doesn't help. The count can be normal one day and zero the next.

What Other Drugs Can Be Used to Treat Hyperthyroidism?

One of the most effective ways to treat hyperthyroidism, when Graves' disease or toxic nodules cause it, is radioactive iodine ablation. Radioactive iodine destroys thyroid cells, which resolves the hyperthyroidism. Because the patient is left with no thyroid, he or she will need to take thyroid hormone replacement for life.

About 90 percent of patients are cured with one dose of radioactive iodine. The purpose of giving radioactive iodine is to destroy (ablate) all of the thyroid permanently.

If you are to have this procedure, you will be instructed to stop taking certain medications ahead of time. Women will be given a pregnancy test since you cannot have this treatment if you are pregnant.

When undergoing radioactive iodine ablation, you are given a pill containing radioactive iodine. The thyroid will absorb most of the radioactive iodine, which it does naturally when extracting iodine from the blood to make hormones. Upon absorption, the radioactive iodine destroys part or all of the thyroid, depending on how much is administered.

You do not need to stay in the hospital. You will be advised to drink lots of fluids to encourage the radioactive iodine to be excreted through your urine. You will be given guidelines to follow once you are treated. The guidelines vary slightly from hospital to hospital.

Radioactive iodine takes several weeks to months to destroy the unwanted tissue, so your doctor may prescribe other medicine to relieve symptoms in the meantime. Without taking other medications, most patients notice their symptoms getting better in about 4 weeks. In 8 to 12 weeks, 60 to 70 percent of patients are cured of hyperthyroidism.

A handful of patients will require a second dose. This is done when symptoms remain after six months. A fraction of patients won't be cured by the second dose and will need surgery.

Radioactive Iodine: Keeping Things Straight. Radioactive iodine is used in a number of ways to diagnose and treat thyroid problems:

1. Radioactive iodine ablation is a treatment for hyperthyroidism caused by Graves' disease. The radioactive iodine is given in a sufficient dose to totally ablate the thyroid, eliminating the problem of hyperthyroidism.

2. Radioactive iodine treatment is not always the same thing as ablation. Radioactive iodine treatment may be used to treat "hot" nodules, which manufacture thyroid hormone independently of the pituitary's orders and may induce hyperthyroidism. In this case, the nodule is destroyed, but the thyroid gland is not ablated and will still produce thyroid hormones. The treatment also may be used to shrink, but not destroy, a goiter. Radioactive tests and treatment are described more in chapter 6, and this particular therapy is described more in chapter 7.

3. Radioactive iodine uptake and scan is a test used to diagnose the cause of hyperthyroidism and provide information about the size and activity of thyroid tissue.

For testing purposes, the patient takes a much smaller dose of radioactive iodine than is used for treatment (20- to 50-fold less). The doctor can measure how much of the iodine the thyroid takes up, which indicates the activity level of thyroid tissue. Then the thyroid is scanned to produce images of the diseased and normal tissues.

As discussed above, a radioactive iodine *uptake and scan* can be used to determine whether a nodule is hot, and then radioactive iodine *treatment* can be used to destroy the hot nodule or ablate the thyroid gland affected by Graves' disease.

Radioactive Iodine Ablation and Women. Pregnant women should not undergo this treatment because the radioactive iodine could destroy the fetus's thyroid and possibly damage its developing tissues. In addition, women who are breast-feeding should not undergo the treatment since the radioactivity will contaminate the breast milk.

Women who have been treated with radioactive iodine should wait 8 to 12 months before conceiving, to avoid any increased risk for congenital defects in the infants.

Radioactive Iodine Ablation and Graves' Disease Patients. Unfortunately, in patients with Graves' disease, it is not possible to give just enough iodine to destroy some of the thyroid and spare the rest so the patient can continue at the right level of thyroid activity. The reason is that the remaining thyroid will continue to be stimulated by the antibodies. It will slowly grow and eventually produce enough hormones to cause a return of hyperthyroidism. Typically, the entire thyroid must be destroyed; then the patient becomes hypothyroid and must take thyroid hormones for the rest of her or his life.

Why Trade Hyperthyroidism for Hypothyroidism?

You may be wondering why anyone would trade hyperthyroidism for hypothyroidism. The fact is, hypothyroidism is much easier and safer to treat over the long term than hyperthyroidism. Graves' can be controlled with antithyroid medications, but as described earlier, every time there is an infection, the patient has to rush to the emergency room.

On the other hand, taking thyroid hormone replacement to treat hypothyroidism is safe, cheap, effective, and easy.

In treating Graves' disease, the dose of radioactive iodine is based on the size of the gland and the results of the uptake test. The larger the gland, the bigger the dose; the higher the uptake, the smaller the dose.

Typically, 150–200 microcuries or 0.15–0.2 millicuries of radioactive iodine are given per gram of thyroid gland. Gland size is determined by physical exam and by experience. An inexperienced physician is less likely to estimate the size accurately.

For example, to destroy a 30-gram thyroid gland would require 30 × 200 microcuries = 6,000 microcuries (6 millicuries). This would be an ideal dose if the entire dose were picked up by the thyroid. But no thyroid gland picks up all the iodine. The radioactive iodine uptake test and scan (see page 98) tells us exactly the proportion that is absorbed.

If the uptake in your thyroid is 50 percent, the radioactive iodine should be doubled, so you would receive 12 millicuries of radioactive iodine. If the uptake is only 30 percent, the dose should be increased to 18 millicuries.

Most of the time, the necessary dose is between 6 and 12 millicuries, but occasionally higher doses are needed. Some physicians use a standard dose for treatment regardless of the test results. This standard dose is typically 10 or 15 millicuries. If the patient is rendered hypothyroid, the treatment is counted as a success. The success rate using a standard dose is just a little worse than when the dose is calculated.

Are There Side Effects with Radioactive Thyroid Ablation?

Many patients' gut reaction is to shun anything with the word *radioactive* attached to it. However, radioactive iodine behaves like a smart bomb: it attacks only the designated target (in this case, the thyroid). Most of the radioactivity is absorbed by the thyroid gland since iodine is routinely picked up only by thyroid cells. In other words, the target attracts the bomb. There is virtually no collateral damage to neighboring tissue. The radioactivity that is not absorbed by the thyroid is quickly eliminated from the body, mostly in the urine.

Some side effects of radioactive thyroid ablation include:

- **Metallic taste.** The most common side effect from radioactive iodine therapy is a metallic taste in the mouth, which lasts a few days to a couple of weeks.

- **Swollen glands.** The second most frequent side effect is swelling of the salivary glands for several days to a couple of weeks. Often, some iodine is absorbed by the salivary glands, which routinely assimilate small amounts of iodine. This may lead to swelling and pain in the jaws and under the tongue. This occurs much more commonly in patients treated for thyroid carcinoma, in whom much larger doses of radioactive iodine are used.

  Preventing this is simple: suck lemon drops to stimulate the saliva flow and wash out the radiation. But wait 24 hours before resorting to lemon drops. If you suck on them the

Side Effects That *Don't* Happen

Some patients fear that absorbing radiation into the thyroid could cause thyroid cancer. Experience has proven otherwise. Over the 50 years of practicing this treatment, hundreds of thousands of hyperthyroid patients have seen success with radioactive iodine, and there has been no evidence of increased incidence of thyroid cancer—or any other type of cancer. However, the monitoring is continuing because we want to be able to detect even a minuscule increase in the risk.

Treatment does not conclusively affect women's or men's reproductive organs, as some patients worry. While there are some reports in the literature describing the occasional male patient who has problems with sperm count after a history of radioactive iodine treatment, doctors are still exploring if this is caused by the treatment. I once had a patient who was treated twice with a high dose of radioactive iodine for thyroid cancer. He was later found to have a complete lack of sperm. We assumed that this was congenital and not related to radioactive iodine treatment. Three years later, he surprised us all, including himself, when he his wife became pregnant. Semen analysis showed complete recovery of his sperm count. Now we think it was related to the radioactive iodine treatments. So we have to stay open-minded and keep learning.

day of treatment, you will activate the salivary cells, which will pick up even more radioactive iodine, intensifying the swelling and pain. After 24 hours, most of the circulating iodine is already excreted from the body, and the salivary cells cannot absorb any additional iodine. The lemon drops can now be used to squeeze out iodine remaining in the salivary gland cells.

- **Vomiting and nausea.** Some patients also experience vomiting and nausea for one or two days after treatment.

A Note for People with Graves' Eye Disease. Radioactive iodine must be used cautiously with patients who have Graves' eye disease. Some studies have shown that the eye disease may worsen after therapy in a small number of patients, especially in patients who smoke.

Can Radioactive Treatments Affect Others Around Me?

If you are planning to have radioactive iodine ablation, here are some crucial guidelines to follow in the days afterward to minimize unnecessary exposure of others to the radiation your body will be carrying until it is completely excreted.

These guidelines are very strict and keep the exposure to others to an absolute minimum. If you consider that people who are *treated* with radioactive iodine have no acute side effects themselves and live 50 years and more with no side effects, it is hard to imagine that someone else would suffer health problems just by being in close proximity. Nonetheless, it is important to follow the guidelines precisely. Better safe than sorry!

Sleeping and Other Close Contact. You should sleep in a separate bed from your spouse or partner for 3 to 12 nights afterward and avoid sexual contact for up to 12 days, depending on the strength of the radioactive iodine dosage.

Close contact with children (hugging, kissing, touching, changing diapers) must be avoided for 3 to 12 days.

You will need to maintain about six feet of space between yourself and others during the first two or three days. During this time, avoid public places, stay home from work for a day or two, and drink plenty of water.

Keeping Your Things Separate. Do not share eating utensils or toothbrushes with family members, and wash these items separately and thoroughly. You should flush the toilet two times after each use, wipe the toilet seat and sink after use, and wash your hands frequently during the first 48 hours.

Shower daily, using separate towels and washcloths. Any clothing you wore during the first two days following treatment should be washed independently of the rest of the laundry.

Protecting Your Baby. Breast-feeding must be discontinued. Both men and women should avoid conception for 8 to 12 months.

In the past, posttreatment safeguards were even stricter, but with our increased understanding of the risks, the precautionary measures have been reduced.

Treating Hyperthyroidism with Surgery

If radioactive iodine fails or patients refuse drug therapy and radioactive iodine, surgery is the other alternative. Surgery cures hyperthyroidism by completely removing the thyroid and, like radioactive iodine ablation, making patients hypothyroid for the rest of their lives.

The operation, called a thyroidectomy, is not considered major surgery. The incision in the neck is small, 2 inches at most. A blood transfusion is not necessary, so there is no risk of being infected by a blood-transmitted disease like HIV or hepatitis C. Also, there is no need to open any important body cavity, which makes the job of the anesthesiologist much easier.

Patients can talk, swallow, eat, drink, and walk immediately after surgery. There is no need to wait months for the treatment to take effect: hyperthyroidism, in most cases, is cured immediately by surgery. The hospital stay is usually just overnight, and you can go back to work whenever you feel comfortable.

Often, hyperthyroidism needs to be controlled before you can have a thyroidectomy because having uncontrolled hyperthyroidism during this surgery puts you at risk for heart problems.

In addition, manipulating a highly overactive gland during surgery could release a deluge of thyroid hormones into the bloodstream, triggering a dangerous thyroid storm (for more on thyroid storms, see page 86).

How Can I Control My Hyperthyroidism Before Surgery?

Usually, hyperthyroidism and its symptoms can be controlled before surgery with antithyroid medications and beta-blockers, but not always. Sometimes patients with large goiters and toxic nodules, in addition to Graves' disease, need to be treated for a week with large doses of elemental (nonradioactive) iodine. This will temporarily block the production and release of thyroid hormones and help control the hyperthyroidism.

Elemental iodine is administered in the form of radiographic contrast agents (such as those used during certain imaging scans). Then a high dose of steroids is given to diminish any inflammation in the gland. This is all done on an outpatient basis.

Patients improve after this therapy, but only temporarily. Surgery must be performed during this period of relative calm—which lasts about a week—or the hyperthyroidism will return and possibly worsen.

Are Thyroidectomies Risky?

The principal danger of surgery is collateral damage to the vocal cord nerves or the parathyroid glands in the neck, which control the body's calcium levels. Accidental damage to the parathyroid glands is rare. When it occurs, it leads to low calcium levels in the blood, which can be temporary or permanent depending on the severity of the damage. The patient may require calcium and vitamin D replacement therapy for life to maintain adequate calcium levels if damage occurs, but again, this rarely happens.

However, damage to one of the vocal cord nerves is more frequent. Although accidentally slicing a vocal cord nerve won't make someone mute, it will change the quality of your voice. Everyone has two vocal chords that vibrate in order to create different sounds when we speak. When one of these nerves is damaged, the paralyzed vocal cord freezes in its position and doesn't vibrate—but it is possible to talk just by using the one remaining vocal cord. Should this happen to you, you will probably sound hoarse and, when singing, will be unable to hit all the notes you could previously.

Thyroidectomies are delicate but not intricate surgeries. Such complications as damaged nerves and glands are not the norm. To avoid such accidents, it is crucial to select a surgeon with experience in operating on thyroids. Always find out how many thyroidectomies the physician performs per year; he or she should perform at least five to ten.

Tracking down an experienced surgeon shouldn't be difficult in major cities, but it can be a challenge in remote areas. It may be worth your while to travel to a large metropolis.

Treating Overactive Nodules

Overactive thyroid nodules, or toxic adenomas, are a much less common cause of hyperthyroidism than Graves' disease. Overactive thyroid nodules are small tumors that acquired the ability to produce thyroid hormones independently of the TSH. Once this happens, the rest of the thyroid goes to sleep because TSH is undetectable, but the patient stays hyperthyroid because the adenomas continue to make hormones.

How Are Toxic Adenomas Treated?

A toxic adenoma (nodule) can be treated with any one of the three options discussed above. However, antithyroid medications are only a temporary measure in these cases; they don't result in a permanent resolution. We generally use them to prepare patients for radioactive iodine treatment or surgery.

Usually, I recommend radioactive iodine ablation rather than surgery for patients with toxic adenomas because it is less invasive, and after treatment, most of these patients will have a normal, healthy thyroid function. In these patients, the toxic nodule is the only operating hormone factory in the body; the pituitary has temporarily closed the normal thyroid factory by halting production of TSH. Therefore, only the tumor absorbs the radioactive iodine. As the toxic nodule slowly dies, the patient's TSH increases, waking up the normal thyroid tissue, which then takes over the production of thyroid hormones, keeping the patient healthy. Only 10 to 20 percent of these patients end up with hypothyroidism after radioactive iodine treatment.

With toxic nodules, dose calculations of radioactive iodine are much more difficult to gauge. Most physicians administer the same dose to all patients. While some doctors use relatively high doses (20–30 millicuries), a recent study showed that 10 millicuries is equally effective.

• • • *Fast Fact* • • •

Toxic nodules are destroyed by radioactive iodine on the first attempt in more than 90 percent of cases.

• • •

Surgery works well too, however. The surgeon will remove only that part of the gland containing the toxic nodule, leaving the rest of the thyroid in place. Afterward, most patients will have normal thyroid function (half a gland is sufficient to supply enough hormone).

Finally, an ethanol (alcohol) injection can be used to treat toxic nodules after preparation with antithyroid medications. This procedure was initially being done only in Europe, but because of its promising results, its use has spread to other parts of the world including the U.S.

How Are Toxic Multinodular Goiters Treated?

Treatment for an enlarged thyroid with multiple nodules producing thyroid hormones is similar to that for toxic nodules. Antithyroid medications are used in the same manner, to calm the symptoms of hyperthyroidism before administering radioactive iodine or surgery.

But treating toxic multinodular goiters requires higher doses of radioactivity and may have a higher incidence of failure than with toxic nodules. About 10 to 15 percent of radioactive iodine treatments fail to normalize the thyroid, so these patients have to be treated again.

Surgery is sometimes the best option for toxic multinodular goiters. And it is the only option for:

- Patients who have both toxic and nontoxic nodules (nodules that don't produce hormones)
- Pregnant patients
- Those for whom radioactive iodine has failed
- Young patients who may want to have children soon
- Patients who have a large goiter exerting pressure on the windpipe or feeding pipe

When it is necessary to resolve the hyperthyroidism quickly, surgery is the best choice because it cures the condition immediately.

Untreated Hyperthyroidism

Sometimes I have a patient with minor hyperthyroid symptoms. For example, she may be slowly losing weight despite a good appetite. When I explain her treatment options, she balks and says, "Why can't I continue like this? I feel pretty good; nothing is seriously bothering me."

I explain that long-term, uncontrolled hyperthyroidism often has serious complications. These include heart arrhythmias (atrial fibrillation is particularly common), cardiac dilation (dilated cardiomyopathy), and even sudden cardiac death. Also, the patient will have bone mineral mass loss, which over time leads to osteoporosis. Therefore, all cases except extremely mild ones will require treatment.

What Is Thyroid Storm?

Thyroid storm is an uncontrollable eruption of thyroid hyperactivity. The hyperactivity of thyroid storm is so intense that medication cannot control the symptoms, and radioactive iodine dangerously worsens symptoms before improving them.

Thyroid storm occurs in untreated or inadequately treated patients and may be triggered by infection, trauma, surgery (not just thyroid surgery), embolism (a clot), diabetic acidosis, uncontrolled diabetes associated with severe metabolic derangement, and complications of pregnancy or labor itself. Symptoms and signs include fever, severe increase in body temperature (hyperpyrexia) with high temperatures from 104 to 106 degrees Fahrenheit, marked weakness and muscle wasting, extreme restlessness with wide emotional swings, confusion, psychosis, and even coma. The liver may be affected, leading to hepatomegaly (liver enlargement) with mild jaundice.

Thyroid storm is a life-threatening emergency. It can kill by causing congestive heart failure, a condition in which the heart cannot pump blood out as strongly as it should. A thyroid storm comes on suddenly and never simply blows over. It must be treated rigorously as soon as it is detected. Fortunately, it is a rare condition today because hyperthyroidism is usually caught and treated as soon as the "storm clouds" begin to gather.

Treating Thyroid Storm. Since thyroid storm is a life-threatening condition, patients need to be admitted into the intensive care unit and treated with supportive measures, such as oxygen (even mechanical ventilation), intravenous fluids containing some sugar (to help the body with its metabolic needs), acetaminophen to lower the temperature, cooling blankets, and ice packs.

Doctors treat thyroid storm by following these measures:

- Heart arrhythmias need to be treated.
- Beta-blockers are used to calm heart symptoms and sleep-related problems.
- Antithyroid drugs are used to stop further production of thyroid hormones.
- Elemental iodine is given to block the release of stored hormones into the bloodstream.
- Steroids are used to block the conversion of T4 to T3.
- Treatment is given for whatever condition triggered the thyroid storm.

If untreated, thyroid storm always leads to death. With successful treatment, symptoms usually improve within 24 hours and are fully controlled in about a week.

Unfortunately, some patients succumb despite adequate treatment. For most, when the storm subsides, a permanent treatment for the hyperthyroidism will be administered, frequently surgery.

In the past, thyroid storm would be triggered when a patient with uncontrolled hyperthyroidism underwent a thyroidectomy without pretreatment. That is why we now control hyperthyroidism before surgery.

Treating Subclinical Hyperthyroidism

Treatment for subclinical hyperthyroidism is controversial. Professional associations such as the American Thyroid Association and the American Association of Clinical Endocrinologists have issued recommendations for screening and treatment, but their recommendations differ.

Until additional scientific data is gathered, treatment decisions must be based on the sound judgment of the practicing physician and the patient's preference.

I believe that treatment should be considered only if the TSH is persistently low and some symptoms of hyperthyroidism appear, such as inability to sleep, fatigue, heart palpitations, weight loss, or anxiety.

In such cases, I use antithyroid medications until the patient's blood tests are normalized. Then I reassess the patient, and if he or she has benefited from normalization of thyroid function (feels better, sleeps better, has more energy, and so on), administering a radioactive iodine uptake and scan allows me to determine the cause of the condition. Afterward, I recommend a long-term treatment.

Chapter 6

Tests for Thyroid Disease

Here is a look at the most common kinds of testing used in thyroid disease. Be aware that there is no such thing as a perfect test, and results should be interpreted in conjunction with a patient's symptoms.

Thyroid-Stimulating Hormone Test

The TSH test is a simple blood test. To date, measuring TSH levels in the bloodstream is the best way to screen for thyroid dysfunction. Why? Because small changes in thyroid hormone levels produce large changes in TSH levels.

As you know, the pituitary-thyroid system works in a kind of feedback loop, like a thermostat. TSH, which is produced in the pituitary gland, regulates hormone production in the thyroid gland. In turn, TSH secretion is controlled by thyroid hormone levels in the blood. Increases and decreases in hormone levels signal the cells in the pituitary to increase or decrease TSH production. Thyroid hormone levels similarly regulate the cells in the hypothalamus that produce thyrotropin-releasing hormone, which is also involved in the regulation of TSH. This means that TSH is very sensitive to hormone fluctuations. The slightest deviations are reflected by the TSH level well before you ever feel symptoms.

Does the TSH Test Have Any Limitations?

The Normal Ranges Can't Be Blindly Applied to Every Patient. The normal TSH range varies slightly from laboratory to laboratory, but in general it is 0.4 to 5.5 microunits per milliliter of blood. Laboratory norms are based on measurements of large groups of people with healthy thyroids. But doctors treat individuals, not groups.

When the TSH of an individual is repeatedly tested, most of the measurements vary about 0.5 microunits per milliliter. If a person's TSH is 1.0 most of the time, in successive tests it will vary from 0.5 to 1.5.

If a person's TSH level is on the high or low end of the normal range, it should not vary so much that it shifts to the opposite end of the spectrum. If this occurs, even though the result is still in the normal range, it may indicate thyroid disease.

The Normal Ranges May Be Off. Recent studies show that when the normal TSH ranges were generated almost 50 years ago, the groups in the tests may have included some people who were mildly hypothyroid and mildly hyperthyroid. Therefore, several professional endocrine societies have advised narrowing the normal range, especially on the high end, from 5.5 to 4.2. Reducing the range will help physicians pick up more people with true thyroid dysfunction who are on the fringes of current normal ranges.

How Should My Doctor Evaluate My TSH Test Results?

Physicians should always take TSH tests with a grain of salt (iodized, preferably!). When used as a screening tool to test people who have no symptoms, a normal result virtually excludes thyroid disease. But with patients who have symptoms suggestive of thyroid dysfunction, the TSH test is only the first step. A doctor should never make a decision based on one number.

Some years ago, a patient was referred to me for hyperthyroidism. The blood test her doctor gave her showed she had a completely suppressed TSH level, a strong indicator of hyperthyroidism. When the woman entered, I was sure she had Graves' disease. She had the classic symptoms: she was visibly shaking and sweating. She was anxious, her muscle mass was gone, and I could see the bones in her arms and shoulders. She wobbled when she entered my office. Also, she had big, prominent eyes and a small goiter that I could see.

Even though I was quite certain of my diagnosis, I repeated the lab tests she had had elsewhere. To my astonishment, her labs came back perfectly normal. Her TSH, T4, and T3 levels were all within a healthy range.

I repeated the tests a few weeks later. They were normal again. She didn't have thyroid disease. Actually, she was suffering from a severe anxiety disorder. I could see her thyroid because she was emaciated, not because she had a goiter.

Her first TSH was probably a lab error. Even the best doctors sometimes get bad lab results—it happens. Again, this is why I never rely on just one test.

What Other Tests Measure Thyroid Hormones?

If a patient's TSH is abnormal, the next step is to measure her thyroid hormones, the T3 and T4 levels in her blood.

T4 and T3 journey through the blood in two ways, either freely or bound to proteins. Only the free T4 and free T3 are active. Thus, physicians are primarily interested in free T4 and free T3.

Calculations. A high free T4 and/or free T3 will indicate hyperthyroidism; a low free T4 and/or free T3 points to hypothyroidism. Until about five or six years ago, lab tests for free thyroid hormone levels were unreliable. Doctors had to measure total T4 (both free and bound T4) and total T3, then make complex calculations to estimate the amounts of free T4 and free T3. (The total T4 test is also known as a serum thyroxine assay; the total T3 test sometimes is referred to as serum triiodothyronine assay.)

But there is a flaw in this method: the measurements can be skewed because some patients have conditions in which the amount of bound T4 is elevated or decreased, while their free T4 level remains normal. For example, we may see an elevation of the bound portion of T4 during pregnancy or when a woman is taking birth control pills or other forms of estrogen. High levels may also occur in some families that are hereditarily prone to have elevated levels of binding proteins. So in these cases, a high total T4 reading does not necessarily indicate hyperthyroidism.

On the other hand, patients with malnutrition have decreased levels of binding proteins in the blood; therefore, their total thyroid hormone levels will be low. Yet again, the free levels will remain normal. As we see, this test isn't always reliable.

Resin Uptake Test. Another way of estimating free T4 levels is by indirectly measuring the levels of binding proteins in the blood using either the T3 or T4 resin uptake test. The estimated amount of binding proteins is multiplied by the total T4 or total T3 (revealed by the total T4 or T3 test). The product (the total T4 multiplied by the amount of binding protein) is called the free T4 index, free thyroxine index (FTI), or sometimes simply T7. This combination of tests is useful in many cases but is not reliable with patients who have extremely high or low levels of thyroid-binding proteins.

More Reliable Tests—Free T4 and Free T3. With the advent of reliable free T4 and free T3 tests, the combination resin uptake and total T4 tests have been falling out of favor. Some general practitioners still rely on these older tests, but most endocrinologists use the simpler and more reliable free thyroid hormone tests.

Low free T4 and/or free T3 could indicate mild thyroid disease even when the TSH is normal. If the TSH is on the high side of normal and free T4 is on the low end, the doctor should be suspicious of hypothyroidism. Similarly, a patient with low TSH, whose free T4 and free T3 are on the high end of normal, may have mild hyperthyroidism.

Together, the TSH test and free T4 and free T3 tests paint an accurate picture of the health of the thyroid. (Nonetheless, sometimes other tests may be needed to determine the precise nature of a patient's condition.)

The free T4 test greatly reduces the confusion related to binding protein abnormalities by taking these abnormalities into account (although, very rarely, there are still some difficulties).

The normal range of free T4 varies with the testing methodology used but is generally between 0.8 and 1.8 nanograms per deciliter.

The free T3 test is another measure of thyroid hormone levels in the blood but is rarely used to diagnose hypothyroidism. Instead, it is frequently used to diagnose hyperthyroidism since some hyperthyroid patients' T4 levels may be deceptively normal while their T3 levels are high. This occurs in T3 toxicosis or T3 hyperthyroidism when patients have toxic nodules that preferentially manufacture T3. A free T4 test would therefore not identify their condition, but a free T3 test would.

• • • *Fast Fact* • • •

The normal free T3 range is
1.8–4.6 nanograms per milliliter.

• • •

Reverse T3 Test. As explained, the body converts T4 into T3 by dislodging one of its four atoms. But the correct atom must be shed. If another is cast off instead, the T4 molecule transforms not into T3, but into reverse T3 (rT3).

Normally, a person converts about 40 percent of his body's T4 into T3 and 60 percent into rT3. If a person becomes sick, fasts, or is highly stressed, these percentages shift: about 20 percent of the available T4 is converted into T3, and the rest is transformed into rT3.

In someone who is healthy, rT3 quickly sloughs off a second atom and transforms into T2 (or diiodothyronine). Then T2 sheds another atom and becomes T1.

A healthy body usually eliminates these molecules within 24 hours. However, serious illnesses block the transformation of rT3 into T2 by inhibiting the enzyme (5'-monodeiodinase) that dislodges the atom. Because of this, patients with serious non-thyroidal illnesses (not including people who have AIDS or kidney failure) have high concentrations of rT3 in their blood.

Some very ill patients may have both low T3 and low TSH, even though they have healthy thyroids. This leads some doctors to suspect that the patient is suffering from a pituitary disorder (low TSH) that may cause hypothyroidism (low T3). Measuring the patient's rT3 levels with a reverse T3 test is helpful in such cases. The rT3 values will be low in patients who are truly hypothyroid because their thyroids will have scaled back T4 production (and T4 provides the raw material for the manufacture of T3 and rT3), but high in patients who have no thyroid condition. Reverse T3 levels are measured by a simple blood test.

Antithyroid Antibody (ATA) Tests

I have already mentioned that we use measurements of antithyroid antibodies to diagnose autoimmune thyroid conditions such are Hashimoto's thyroiditis and Graves' disease. In both of these conditions, the patient's immune system mistakenly mounts an attack on thyroid tissue. In the course of the attack these antibodies are produced, and we can use them to detect the presence of the disease.

What Kinds of Antibodies Are There?

Microsomal Antibody Test. This test has many names: thyroid antimicrosomal antibody, antimicrosomal antibody, microsomal antibody, and thyroid peroxidase antibody. Don't be confused—they are all the same blood test!

The immune system produces microsomal antibodies that are aimed at components of the thyroid cells. Microsomal antibodies themselves are not damaging to the thyroid cells, but presence of these antibodies signifies ongoing thyroid damage that may lead to hypothyroidism (specifically Hashimoto's thyroiditis). The immune system attack on the thyroid also consists of deployment of an army of immune cells, or lymphocytes. These cells travel into the thyroid gland and directly damage thyroid cells. Microsomal antibodies are a side product of the attack and are not damaging themselves. However, it is easy to measure them, while there is no practical way to detect lymphocytes directed to thyroid tissue. The microsomal antibody test detects the presence and measures the level of microsomal antibodies.

Four percent of patients with increased levels of microsomal antibodies become hypothyroid within a year. Then more and more patients develop full-blown hypothyroidism every year thereafter. Yet primary care physicians rarely test for antithyroid microsomal antibodies when the TSH is normal, partly because insurance companies balk at paying for what they deem unnecessary testing.

I use this test when the TSH and free T4 and T3 are normal, but the patient appears to be on the verge of hypothyroidism. I also use this test to confirm or exclude Hashimoto's thyroiditis. I think it is important to check whether antibodies are present as I decide whether to offer treatment or just have the patient come back in

six months for a follow-up. Once I find positive microsomal antibodies, it is rarely necessary to check them again. This is because the
antibodies are just a marker of the disease and by themselves do not
cause any symptoms. The damage to the thyroid cells is inflicted by
immune cells that infiltrate thyroid tissue. Thus, there is no useful
information that can be derived from repeating this test.

Once the antibodies are being produced, repeating the tests
will find them positive for decades after the onset of the disease.
Once the whole thyroid is destroyed, the antibodies may slowly
disappear from the circulation.

Antithyroglobulin Antibody Test. Thyroglobulin is a large protein molecule produced exclusively by thyroid cells. The antithyroglobulin antibody (TgAb) test may indicate Hashimoto's
thyroiditis by detecting abnormally high levels of antithyroglobulin antibodies, which attack thyroglobulin proteins in the thyroid
in this disease. But most doctors who suspect Hashimoto's prefer using the microsomal antibody test because it is a more sensitive indicator. In the beginning of Hashimoto's thyroiditis, the
immune system tends to make more antithyroglobulin antibodies,
but with time it starts making more microsomal antibodies and
stops making antithyroglobulin antibodies. Once the patient has
already developed hypothyroidism, it is more likely to see microsomal antibodies (and a positive microsomal antibody test) than
antithyroglobulin antibodies.

On the other hand, the antithyroglobulin antibody test is always
administered after thyroid cancer surgery in conjunction with a
thyroglobulin test (see page 104). The antithyroglobulin antibody
test is given as a follow-up to confirm the results of the thyroglobulin test and see whether or not these results can be trusted. If the
thyroglobulin antibody test is positive, the test for thyroglobulin
itself cannot be trusted. This is because the antibodies against thyroglobulin interfere with measurement and make the results falsely
low. Measurement of the thyroglobulin is important in patients

with thyroid cancer because absence of thyroglobulin indicates that it has been cured and its presence indicates either persistence of the disease or return of cancer after the cure.

About 20 to 30 percent of thyroid cancer patients have antithyroglobulin antibodies. These patients need whole body radioactive iodine scans to check for recurrence of cancer since thyroglobulin tests aren't reliable (see chapter 8).

Thyroid Receptor Antibody Test. Thyroid receptor antibodies attach to the cell receptors where TSH normally docks. As you may recall from chapter 4, the antibodies pose as TSH, tricking the receptors so that they signal the cells to produce more T4 and T3, causing hyperthyroidism. High levels of the stimulating form of these antibodies (thyroid-stimulating antibodies) are a strong indication that a patient has Graves' disease.

The thyroid receptor antibodies test (a blood test) should be administered if the patient's TSH is suppressed or on the low end of the normal range. This helps us to determine whether Graves' disease is the cause of the suppressed TSH.

Not all thyroid receptor antibodies pose as TSH; some actually block TSH action after attaching to the receptors. These are called thyroid-blocking antibodies, and they usually represent a small portion of the total thyroid receptor antibodies. But on rare occasions, they are the majority and block so much TSH that they actually cause hypothyroidism.

Nuclear Medicine Scans and Tests

Let's start with a quick overview of nuclear medicine since this is the department where the next group of tests is done.

In nuclear medicine, a small amount of radioactive material, such as an iodine isotope, is either swallowed by mouth or injected into the patient. The substance emits gamma rays from inside the body, wherever its target organ is. The rays are detected by a special gamma camera that feeds information to a computer, which then translates the data into images of the organ.

Rather than drawing a shadow image of an organ (like an X-ray), gamma rays show us how an organ is functioning. They allow us to see how the organ—in this case, the thyroid—accumulates and excretes the radioactive material.

The radiation levels used in nuclear medicine are lower than what a patient receives from an X-ray or CT scan, so they are very safe. The same precautions we discussed in the section on radioactive iodine treatments, for example, are unnecessary when you submit to these tests.

What Is a Radioactive Iodine Uptake Test and Scan?

The dynamic duo of diagnostic thyroid tests is known as a radioactive iodine uptake test and scan. This name describes exactly what it is: the measurement of the amount of radioactive iodine that the thyroid takes up (absorbs) and, next, a scan of the thyroid.

This combination of tests is extremely useful in helping doctors determine the cause of hyperthyroidism and the dose of radioactive iodine necessary to treat Graves' disease and thyroid cancer.

Studies of the thyroid gland are done with radioactive iodine. This usually raises the question: why radioactive and why iodine? The second part of the question has a quicker answer than the first part, so let's start there.

If you remember that the thyroid naturally absorbs iodine, you'll understand why it is a useful substance when we want to know more about whether the thyroid is functioning properly. We can measure whether the thyroid absorbs a normal or abnormal amount of iodine in a given period.

As for the radioactivity, it supplies the gamma rays that allow for detection of iodine from outside the body using a gamma camera. This signal is then used to measure how much iodine is taken up and to obtain images of the thyroid to see whether there are abnormalities such as nodules or tumors. (See page 100 for more information on why gamma rays work in scanning.)

For seven to ten days before this test, you'll need to stop taking any antithyroid medications (such as PTU or Tapazole) so that the blockade of thyroid hormone synthesis is stopped and true measurements can be obtained. On the day of the test, you will swallow a pill containing a small, safe amount of radioactive iodine. The particular type of radioactive isotope will be iodine-131 or iodine-123.

Then there is a waiting period, usually about four hours, during which the iodine collects in the thyroid. After the wait is over, the technician will check how much iodine the thyroid has picked up. This is the uptake portion of the test. It is done while you lie still, on your back, and a scanner detects where the iodine has gathered and how intense the gamma rays coming from it are. The procedure is painless. Some hospitals require a 24-hour wait until the uptake. This allows for measurements that are somewhat more precise, but it may be less convenient for patients, who will have to come in on two consecutive days.

The amount of radioactive iodine the thyroid absorbs tells us whether or not the gland is functioning normally. If the thyroid absorbs more than a normal amount, it is overactive, or hyperthyroid. If it picks up very little, the thyroid is underactive, or hypothyroid.

In the United States, a normal thyroid gland picks up between 9 and 15 percent of the dose in four hours. This uptake range varies, depending on how much iodine there is in circulation, which in turn depends on how much iodine individuals consume in their diet.

If a patient has Graves' disease, a large portion of the iodine will be absorbed (typically, 40 to 80 percent). But in cases of thyroiditis or accidental or intentional ingestion of thyroid hormones, the uptake will be very low (0 to 9 percent).

After the uptake portion, while you continue lying down, the gamma ray camera will scan your thyroid to obtain a picture of the gland. This will show the distribution of the iodine inside the thyroid and whether there are any nodules or other abnormalities.

Why Do Gamma Rays Work in Scanning?

Like rambunctious teenagers, radioactive isotopes bristle with unstable energy that they throw off in all directions. Radioactive substances emit this excess energy in three forms: as alpha rays, beta rays, or gamma rays—or a combination of these.

These rays are like three types of teens: alpha rays are bulky, slow adolescents who clumsily collide with everything around them; beta rays are midsized, very aggressive teens that attack everything they encounter; and gammas are like a pint-sized Speedy Gonzales who can slip past anything.

Positively charged alpha rays are too big to penetrate the skin—even a sheet of paper or the outer layer of human skin stops them in their tracks. They can't do any external damage, but once they infiltrate the body (via an injected or ingested alpha emitter), alpha rays wreak havoc on cell structure, but only in the immediate vicinity of where they are emitted. They are too big and slow to move around much. After smashing up the neighborhood, alphas are too tired to do any more harm. So they stabilize and turn into helium.

• • • Fast Fact • • •

Alpha rays fly at only one-twentieth the speed of light, compared to gamma rays, which travel at the speed of light.

• • •

The negatively charged beta rays are faster and have much more endurance than alphas. They are small enough to penetrate the skin, and once inside the body, they cover a lot more ground than alpha rays. Therefore, the damage they inflict is more widely dispersed. However, the distance they travel in the soft tissue is still very short, ranging from one-fifteenth to one-tenth of an inch.

Gamma rays are the roadrunners of the radioactive gang. They are pure energy and carry no charge (no positive or negative attitude). Gamma particles are so tiny, they can penetrate anything and tend to speed past organs and tissue in their lightning-fast journey through the body. They don't often bump or run into things like their bigger cousins. Because of their ability to penetrate flesh, bone, and even lead shields, gamma rays are ideal for scanning.

After unleashing all their volatile energy by emitting alpha, beta, and/or gamma rays, radioactive substances settle down (or stabilize) and live the quiet life (like middle-aged people compared to teenagers). They become nonradioactive elements such as carbon, lead, helium, or oxygen.

What Will a Gamma Ray Scan Reveal?

Gamma ray scans provide a picture of the distribution of radioactive iodine in the gland by detecting gamma rays emanating from its atoms. If a patient has Graves' disease, the entire thyroid will pick up the radioactive iodine, and the scan will show a smooth, even distribution of iodine. The entire bow tie of the thyroid will be visible.

If the patient is hyperthyroid because of a tumor that autonomously manufactures thyroid hormone, only the tumor will absorb the radioactive iodine, and only the tumor will show up on the scan. As you may remember, this is because, in hyperthyroidism, the pituitary halts TSH production, virtually shutting down the thyroid factory; therefore, the thyroid will not absorb any radioactive iodine to manufacture hormones.

If the patient has thyroiditis, the bow tie will be barely visible or completely invisible because the thyroid will take up virtually no iodine; the pituitary has closed it down in response to the deluge of reserve hormones spilling into the bloodstream. (Remember that thyroiditis punctures holes in the thyroid warehouses, allowing reserve hormones to leak into the blood.) Also, inside an inflamed thyroid, the cells are damaged and have great difficulty picking up any iodine.

If a patient has ingested thyroid hormone inadvertently or intentionally—by eating cow thyroids in hamburger, for example—the scan will look exactly like thyroiditis because the excess of thyroid hormone signals the pituitary to halt production of TSH and suspend hormone production in the thyroid factory.

When the bow tie is invisible and the doctor suspects the patient has been ingesting thyroid hormone on the sly, a second test called a thyroglobulin assay must be administered to ascertain whether the patient has thyroiditis or has in fact ingested thyroid hormone.

Are There Different Forms of Radioactive Iodine?

There are several isotopes of radioactive iodine. An isotope is a variant of an element. It has the same number of electrons and protons as the corresponding element but a different number of neutrons. Some isotopes are radioactive; others are not.

In thyroid medicine, we use radioactive iodine isotopes such as I-123, I-124, I-125, and I-131. The designations such as "123" represent the isotope's atomic weight. The "123" means there are a total of 123 protons and neutrons in the isotope. The weight of the much smaller electrons is negligible.

If you are having a radioactive iodine uptake and scan, you will probably be given radioactive iodine I-123 or I-131. Iodine-125 is used in laboratory medicine for a variety of blood tests. Nonradioactive iodine-127 is the iodine found in nature.

Some iodine isotopes emit gamma rays, while others emit both beta and gamma rays. Iodine-123 is ideal for scanning because it emits only gamma rays. The energy of this gamma ray is 159 kiloelectron volts, which is nearly ideal for today's gamma cameras. Unfortunately, it is significantly more expensive than I-131.

Iodine-131, much cheaper, can be—and frequently is—used for scanning. However, its gamma ray energy is 384 kiloelectron volts, which is not ideal for the cameras. Iodine-131 also emits beta rays, which may damage tissue, and it is not useful for scanning because once inside the body, the rays cannot escape it. Because of the beta ray, the dose that is given is limited and smaller than when I-123 is used.

Although iodine-131's beta rays are a drawback in scanning, they are an advantage in treatment. These beta rays are electrons that spray or radiate in all directions from atoms. When a large number of beta rays pass through the body, their energy is absorbed by the tissue they encounter. The molecular structure of this tissue is broken up and the tissue destroyed.

Iodine-131 is the only isotope used to treat thyroid disease. Its beta ray energy is about 190 kiloelectron volts. It can penetrate soft tissue anywhere from 0.6 millimeters to 2.0 millimeters deep.

Since the thyroid cells naturally import iodine from the bloodstream to manufacture thyroid hormone, they absorb and concentrate iodine-131 up to 40 times higher than the levels in circulation. The damage inflicted by I-131 beta rays, therefore, is primarily concentrated in the thyroid or nodule, destroying the tissue that is causing the patient's problem. The rest of the body receives very little radiation.

Radioactive iodine treatment allows physicians to deliver huge amounts of radiation to the thyroid while sparing the rest of the body. No other radiation therapy can achieve such precision of delivery.

Iodine-131 decays or loses its radioactivity relatively fast. Half of the radioactivity decays every eight days. In several weeks, it all dissipates.

Why Don't Doctors Always Use Radioactive Iodine Tests if They're So Great?

Although the radioactive iodine test is very useful for pinpointing thyroid problems, it cannot always be used. If a patient's body has been loaded with iodine from other sources, radioactive iodine will be outnumbered (outcompeted) and will not make its way to the thyroid.

For example, patients taking amiodarone will not benefit from the radioactive iodine uptake test because that particular drug already contains large amounts of iodine. Also, patients who have recently had a CT scan in which contrast was used will not be candidates because the radiologic contrast is made largely of iodine.

Finally, women who are pregnant should not undergo any procedures involving ingestion of radioactive material. Nursing mothers should be sure to discuss the risks of this procedure with their physician before proceeding.

What Is a Thyroglobulin Test?

If a radioactive iodine test shows very low uptake, the thyroid's overactivity could be caused by a number of conditions: thyroiditis, unintentional or intentional ingestion of thyroid hormone, or struma ovarii or some other ectopic thyroid tumor. We use the thyroglobulin test to ascertain which of these conditions the patient has.

Thyroglobulin is the protein chain used to manufacture T3 and T4. Large amounts of it are stored in the thyroid follicles.

Normally, the thyroglobulin level is from 2 to 22 nanograms per milliliter. If the thyroglobulin level is extremely high, we know the patient has thyroiditis since thyroiditis spills thyroglobulin into the bloodstream.

If the level is undetectable, the patient has probably ingested thyroid hormone. In this case, the thyroid will "sleep" and not release any thyroglobulin.

On the other hand, if the thyroglobulin level is normal, the patient's hyperthyroidism may be caused by an autonomous thyroid tumor.

A thyroglobulin test is also the best indicator of cancer relapse in patients who have had thyroid cancer. After cancer surgery, there should be no thyroglobulin in the body, so the test should be negative. If the thyroglobulin level becomes positive again, we know the cancer has returned.

What Is PET Imaging?

Positron emission tomography (PET) imaging is the newest and most expensive imaging process.

First, you are given an intravenous solution, and within an hour you are scanned. You lie on a gurney that is slid gently into the center of a machine with a large ringed detector; it is almost as if you are in the center of a giant doughnut. The scan usually lasts less than an hour.

How the Scan Is Generated. A positron is a positively charged electron. Electrons are normally negative, and positrons (which are their opposite) are called antimatter or antielectrons. Such particles cannot exist in our universe except for exceedingly short periods.

As positrons emanate from an atom, they are immediately attracted by the closest electron (opposite charges attract each other). When positrons and electrons meet or collide, they annihilate each other, converting into pure energy. Their collision produces two gamma rays (the energy of which is 511 kiloelectron volts each), which travel in exact opposite directions. The necklace of detectors surrounding the patient picks up these rays.

Finally, a computer generates a picture of the body tissue from which the gamma rays emanate. The newest machines also perform a simultaneous CT scan. They provide a combination picture that consists of a whole body CT scan fused with the PET scan. This enables the physician to see exactly where the PET signal is located in the body.

PET imaging is especially useful in pinpointing recurring thyroid cancers and many other cancers. Often, positron emission tomography will ferret out disease sites that I-131 scans cannot.

The most commonly used positron-emitting isotope is fluorine-18. This isotope can be incorporated into the glucose (sugar) molecule to form fluorodeoxyglucose (FDG). This form of glucose will be absorbed by cells but cannot be used for energy production like normal glucose. Therefore, it gets stranded in the cells, where it can be detected by the PET scanner. Since malignant tumors have a high metabolism, they pick up much more fluorodeoxyglucose than normal tissue and thereby reveal their location.

The other isotope used to detect thyroid cancer with PET is iodine-124. However, I-124 use is only investigational at this time. I expect that it will play a more important role in the future.

Testing the Lumps

Nodules and lumps can sometimes be discovered during a physical exam, but an ultrasound examination is the best way to characterize them. This safe and painless test has been in use for years.

An ultrasound machine generates an ultrasound pulse that passes from the handheld transducer or probe through a gel into the patient's neck. When the sound wave bumps into a border between tissues, a change in the density of the surface, it bounces back to the probe. A computer then draws a picture based on these reflected sound waves.

An ultrasound examination can detect very small structures, such as blood vessels and even the tiniest thyroid nodules (2 to 3 millimeters in size). Ultrasound also helps determine whether a nodule is a cyst (filled with fluid) or a solid mass, or it can indicate that a nodule may be cancerous.

Physicians can measure and monitor the growth rate of nodules with periodic ultrasound tests. Rapidly growing nodules, those containing calcifications inside the nodule (not around the nodule), and those with irregular borders are more likely to be cancerous.

Ultrasound can also detect movement inside the body. This allows us to see where the blood is flowing and how much blood flow there is. The thyroid nodules that show more blood flow than normal thyroid tissue are also more likely to be cancerous.

Finally, the latest development in the field of ultrasound thyroid examination is measurement of the hardness of the nodules. This is called elastography, and it employs the ability of the ultrasound to measure deformation of the nodule under pressure. Cancerous nodules are generally harder than benign nodules and normal thyroid tissue. This method still needs to be validated in a real clinical arena.

Nodules larger than 1 centimeter that don't produce thyroid hormones (cold nodules) or that exhibit features suggestive of cancer on an ultrasound should be biopsied.

What Is a Biopsy and How Is It Done?

A biopsy is a test that takes suspicious tissue from the body so it can be examined under a microscope. For the thyroid, this is done with a needle, usually using a fine needle aspiration.

Fine Needle Aspiration (FNA). This biopsy is performed with a thin needle (the same size that is used for blood tests or smaller). The physician inserts the needle into the nodule and draws (aspirates) a small quantity of cells from it. If the lump is relatively small, the physician may use ultrasound to help guide the needle into the nodule. The cells are examined under a microscope to determine whether they are cancerous or not.

Most physicians performing FNA place the needle twice into each nodule to obtain enough material for a diagnosis. Some doctors first apply a local anesthetic to numb the skin before aspiration. However, I find that it takes two needle sticks just to apply the anesthetic to numb the skin, which can be more painful than the FNA. Because of this, I usually don't use local anesthetic. Instead, I apply an ice cube (tucked inside the examination glove) to the part of the neck where the needle will be applied. This is usually sufficient to numb the skin.

After the needle is removed from the nodule, a small amount of the extracted material is smeared on a microscopic slide, and the rest is washed into a preserving solution. This must be done immediately to prevent any drying of the cells. Once the extracted material is in the solution, it can be preserved without degradation of the cells, allowing time for it to get to the pathologist.

The fine needle aspiration biopsy yields four possible results:

1. The nodule is benign. This occurs in about 80 to 85 percent of cases. Nevertheless, benign nodules need to be periodically rechecked by ultrasound to see whether or not they've grown.

2. The nodule is suspicious for cancer. About 12 to 15 percent of biopsied nodules fall into this category. There are two subgroups in this category. If the FNA indicates that the tumor is a follicular neoplasm, follicular cancer cannot be ruled out; 15 percent of follicular neoplasms eventually prove to be cancers. But sometimes the FNA indicates that the nodule is suspicious for papillary thyroid cancer. Most of these nodules prove to be cancer. In any case, surgery is needed to find out.

3. Cancer cells are found in the biopsy, at which point the physician will recommend treatment.

4. The biopsy is sometimes classified as nondiagnostic. This means that not enough tissue was removed to make a diagnosis. This happens in about 2 to 5 percent of biopsies.

If a biopsy is nondiagnostic, the procedure should be repeated. If, after a second biopsy, the result is still nondiagnostic, most endocrinologists will not attempt a third biopsy but will simply monitor the nodule for growth using ultrasound.

Coarse Needle Biopsy (CNB). In a coarse needle biopsy, also called a cutting-needle biopsy, a larger hollow needle is used to draw out a small cylinder-shaped core of tissue from the lump. The needle is 1 millimeter in diameter or larger.

Besides providing information about individual cells, a coarse needle biopsy helps us understand the architectural pattern and connections between cells (unlike FNA, which shows only a lump of cells that are removed without maintaining their relationship to one another).

To use a coarse needle biopsy, the nodule must be at least 1.5 centimeters, about three-quarters of an inch.

The range of results is very similar to those of FNA. Some studies show that patients who have had a coarse needle biopsy are less likely to undergo surgery than those who have not had this type of biopsy because it might be a little bit more accurate.

Hence, a coarse needle biopsy may yield more accurate results, but it is a more difficult procedure. This is especially true when the nodule is very low in the neck or when a patient is obese. Also, because the needle is large, there is a higher, albeit very small, risk (less than 1 percent) of bleeding and of injury to the windpipe or nerves supplying the vocal cords. Most endocrinologists do not use this technique.

I hope this chapter made some sense of the tests we use to diagnose thyroid disorders, assess the severity before treatment, and guide us in our treatment decisions.

Chapter 7

Nodules and Goiters

I n this chapter, we will explore types and symptoms of nodules and goiters.

Nodules

Thyroid nodules are lumps in the thyroid gland. They are very common, occurring in perhaps half the world's population. Most thyroid nodules are abnormal growths or tumors, and some are cysts (fluid-filled spaces in the tissue), although even the tumors may have cystic components. Most thyroid nodules cause no symptoms whatsoever, are small, and are detectable only by imaging techniques like ultrasound, CT, or MRI. Fortunately, most nodules are benign, but about 5 percent are cancerous.

Generally, women are much more susceptible to developing thyroid nodules than men are, especially after age 60. In fact, 50 to 75 percent of women grow one or more nodules in their lifetimes. However, nodules in men are more likely to be cancerous.

Nodules develop either as single lumps or in clusters called multinodular goiters. Single nodules are more likely to be cancerous than multinodular goiters are.

Who Has Nodules?

- One in 12 to 15 women under age 30 has a thyroid nodule.
- One in 40 men under age 30 has a thyroid nodule.
- Half of all people will develop a thyroid nodule by the time they are 50.
- The incidence of thyroid nodules increases with age.
- 50 percent of 50-year-olds will have at least one thyroid nodule.
- 60 percent of 60-year-olds will have at least one thyroid nodule.
- 70 percent of 70-year-olds will have at least one thyroid nodule.

Although nodules in children develop far less frequently than in adults, they are four times more likely to be cancerous.

Since most nodules exhibit no symptoms or signs, a large portion of them go undetected. Small nodules are usually discovered by accident, through imaging scans for other conditions. Doctors also discover nodules simply by feeling patients' necks during routine physical exams. Nodules can be felt before they can be seen.

Visible nodules may be noticed while putting on makeup or shaving, or by family or friends.

When found, larger nodules need to be checked to rule out even mild hyperthyroidism or thyroid cancer. Because of this, it is important to have your neck periodically examined.

Daniel Soric

A lump in the throat stood between Daniel Soric and the career he had been preparing for all his life. In August 2002, the shortest man in Croatian volleyball was poised to sign a $1 million, three-year contract with an elite Italian team. The diminutive Soric is five foot four, 127 pounds.

But during a routine pre-signing physical, team doctor Andrej Dupsic discovered a large lump in Soric's throat, just under the Adam's apple. The doctor suspected a thyroid nodule and believed it might be cancerous.

Soric's contract and possibly his career as a volleyball setter were on the line. But Soric had dodged obstacles all his life. To him, a thyroid nodule, even a malignant one, was just one more opponent to outmaneuver.

Soric hadn't seen or felt any problems before, but at his doctor's insistence, Soric flew to see me at the Cleveland Clinic. I had known his family in Croatia, where I grew up and studied medicine, so it was nice to see him again.

After examining him, both the pathologist and I strongly suspected that the nodule was cancerous. It was 6 centimeters—that's a pretty big nodule—and it was harder than normal. I biopsied it with a fine needle aspiration biopsy.

In two hours, the results came back. The nodule was suspicious for cancer.

I told him we had to remove it immediately. The next day in the early morning, the nodule and half of Soric's thyroid were excised. Surgery lasted one and half hours. I saw him in the hospital room in the afternoon and he felt good. He had only a minimal tenderness over the small incisions in the neck, but his voice was strong. He kept his cool while asking me about surgery. I told him that we needed to wait for the final pathology report, and if suspicion of the cancer was confirmed, he would need to have the rest of his thyroid removed.

When the pathologist examined the tissue from Soric's nodule under the microscope, he discovered that it was benign. Nevertheless, removing large, hard nodules is standard practice; they can continue to grow and eventually become malignant.

Soric was relieved and only then admitted how worried he had been. I explained that the half of the thyroid gland remaining in his neck would be perfectly able to provide him all the thyroid hormones he needed and he did not need to take any medications. However, I advised him to have his neck examined by his regular physician from time to time to monitor for any new nodules.

A few months later, I got an email from his doctor saying Soric's TSH was 6.7 and he wasn't feeling as energetic as he used to. It turns out his remaining thyroid was not quite enough to keep him perfectly healthy. I advised the doctor to start Soric on thyroid hormone and adjust his dose until his TSH was below 2.0 microunits per milliliter.

Just as he expected, Soric outflanked the lump in his neck— with an assist from modern medicine. He quickly rebounded from surgery and then signed the contract with the Italian team.

Now, like Harry Potter, Soric has a scar to remind him of his fateful encounter. He takes thyroid medication like millions of other people, but he is healthy. Rated as one of the top setters in Europe, Daniel Soric continues to be among the giants of volleyball.

How Many Different Types of Nodules Are There?

There are five types of nodules.

Colloid Nodules. Colloid nodules make up 70 percent of all nodules. These benign tumors have well-defined follicles, each containing a colloid or protein pool (thus the name colloid nodule).

A patient may have one or many of these nodules. Although colloid nodules can grow quite large, they never spread beyond the thyroid.

Follicular Adenomas. Follicular adenomas consist of many small follicles called microfollicles, but their interior is empty, as if the protein pool had been drained. These are also benign nodules, but it is very difficult to distinguish between follicular adenomas and their malignant cousin, follicular cancer, based only on the cells obtained by thyroid biopsy. Out of 100 follicular neoplasms (the umbrella term used to describe both follicular adenomas and follicular cancers), 15 percent will be cancerous.

Follicular cancer cells are hard to identify because they don't conform to the general rule of how malignant cells should look under a microscope. Malignant cells usually have a mixed appearance, as opposed to cells in benign tumors, which are roughly the same size and look alike.

Follicular cancer cells don't follow this rule of thumb. They fake us out because they look like benign tumor cells; their structure is uniform. Because of this, every follicular adenoma must be surgically removed and examined to be absolutely sure it is not cancerous.

This type of surgery lasts from 90 minutes to four hours and is done under general anesthesia. As long as there are no complications, the patient can expect an overnight stay in the hospital.

After the surgery, a pathologist examines the tumor, looking for invasive cancer cells. These are cells that smash through blood vessel walls and infiltrate the bloodstream, or cells that invade through the outer capsule of the nodule. Because of this action, we can tell that they are malignant, not benign.

Unfortunately, at present we have no better tool than surgery to distinguish between benign and malignant follicular neoplasms.

Thyroid Cysts. Thyroid cysts are fluid-filled lumps. Some are simple cysts made only of fluid and are usually benign. Others are complex cysts composed of both fluid and solid matter that grows from the cell walls. These are more likely to be cancerous.

Inflammatory Nodules. Inflammatory nodules can be caused by chronic inflammation (thyroiditis), or they may occur after pregnancy. These nodules can frequently be recognized by ultrasound and require no further evaluation. Usually, they disappear when inflammation quiets down.

Cancerous Nodules. Cancerous nodules are usually hard and can be quite large (3 centimeters or more), which is why I suspected Daniel Soric's nodule was malignant.

Although most nodules are benign, you may be at risk for developing a cancerous one if you have a family history of thyroid cancer or other forms of endocrine gland cancer, have had neck or head radiation to treat acne or other conditions of the face or head, or are under 20 or over 60 and have a large, hard nodule.

What Causes Nodules?

The cause of nodules is still unknown, but there are risk factors that make some people predisposed to them. These include:

- A family history of benign thyroid nodules

- A shortage of iodine in the diet

- A preexisting thyroid condition, such as Hashimoto's or Graves' disease

Another group of people at risk are those who were treated with radiation therapy for acne, birthmarks, ringworm of the scalp, whooping cough, enlarged thymus, or enlarged adenoids or tonsils. In the 1920s through the early 1960s, between one and two million Americans were given this type of radiation therapy as children. (Such therapies have since been abandoned.)

Anyone affected by fallout from the 1986 Chernobyl nuclear accident or from atomic-bomb testing in the Marshall Islands is at higher than normal risk for developing nodules and thyroid cancer, as are survivors of the Hiroshima and Nagasaki bombings.

What Are the Symptoms of Thyroid Nodules and Multinodular Goiters?

Thyroid nodules are almost always asymptomatic but occasionally can cause mechanical symptoms. For example, if the nodule obstructs the esophagus (food pipe), patients may experience difficulty swallowing food or water. A nodule may also press against the windpipe (trachea), obstructing breathing. However, this happens rarely and patients who have such symptoms do not usually have a thyroid nodule; the problem is usually caused by something else. For a thyroid nodule to cause this kind of symptom, it has to be large and also be at least partially positioned behind the breast bone. Behind the bone, there is no room to expand but backwards, which compresses the feeding and breathing pipe.

Listed below are all the possible symptoms, but almost all of them are rare. When present, the possibility of malignant disease should be seriously considered:

- There is pressure-like sensation when swallowing.
- There is discomfort when tying a tie or buttoning a top button.
- There is pain from bleeding inside the nodule.
- If the nodule is putting pressure on the jugular veins, veins in the neck and face will be distended.
- Transient or permanent paralysis of the nerve that enters into the voice box and innervate vocal cords may cause hoarseness.
- The nerve input to the diaphragm (main breathing muscle) may also be paralyzed, but this is very rare.
- Pressure on the nerve centers in the neck that control involuntary functions of the eye can cause Horner's syndrome, a condition that causes the upper eyelid to droop and the pupil of the affected eye to shrink. Also, sweating is inhibited on that side of the face.

Elderly people are more likely to experience difficulty swallowing or breathing, as they are more likely to have a large multinodular goiter that is growing downward into the chest cavity. These goiters, known as substernal goiters, exert pressure on the trachea (windpipe) and/or the esophagus. Coughing occurs in 10 to 30 percent of patients when the goiter grows under the breastbone. Since they are located behind the breastbone, ultrasound, which cannot penetrate bone, is unable to detect them. A CT scan or an MRI must be used to identify a substernal goiter.

What Does It Mean to Say a Nodule Is Hot or Cold?

Once we find a nodule, we must determine whether it is hot or cold. A hot (or toxic) nodule manufactures thyroid hormone independently of the pituitary's orders and may induce hyperthyroidism, but it is virtually never cancerous. Cold nodules do not produce hormone, but they are more likely to be malignant.

One way to tell whether the nodule is hot is by checking the TSH. If it is low or suppressed, the nodule might be hot (since the thyroid hormone that the nodule produces signals the pituitary to curtail TSH production). If the TSH is normal or elevated, the nodule is cold.

To determine if a nodule is hot or cold, the patient must have a radioactive iodine uptake test and scan to confirm that the nodule is hot and to rule out Graves' disease. A hot nodule will show a high concentration of radioactive iodine on the scan.

If the original TSH test found a cold nodule, the patient does not need to have a radioactive iodine uptake test and scan. Nonetheless, sometimes a cold nodule will show up on this test. For example, if a person with an otherwise overactive thyroid gland had a radioactive iodine scan and test, and the patient had a cold nodule present in the gland, the entire thyroid would uniformly pick up the radioactive iodine except for the nodule area, which is then seen as a cold area in the scan.

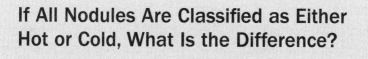

If All Nodules Are Classified as Either Hot or Cold, What Is the Difference?

Hot Nodules (also called toxic)

- Manufacture thyroid independently of the pituitary's orders
- May induce hyperthyroidism
- Are virtually never cancerous

Cold Nodules

- Do not produce hormone
- Do not affect overall thyroid function
- Are more likely to be malignant

How Do You Treat a Hot Nodule?

The treatment of hot nodules may include radioactive iodine ablation, antithyroid medications, injection of alcohol into the nodule, or thyroidectomy. More details on these can be found in chapter 5 and later in this chapter.

How Do You Treat a Cold Nodule?

Before deciding how to treat a cold nodule, the doctor must know how large it is. This is done by using ultrasound. If the nodule is less than 1 centimeter and appears to be benign, the physician will simply monitor it with ultrasound to see if it grows. Follow-up ultrasound examinations should be administered in six months, then again in one year.

If a cold nodule is larger than 1 centimeter in diameter, we need to find out whether it is cancerous or not. Usually, this is done with FNA biopsy. Sometimes I will perform the biopsy on the nodule that is smaller than 1 centimeter in diameter. This is the case if the nodule reveals some worrisome features during the ultrasound examination. If the nodule has an irregular border, increased blood flow, or if it contains small grains of calcifications inside itself, I would opt for FNA biopsy. On the other hand, sometimes I will not perform a biopsy even if the nodule is larger than 1 centimeter in size. This is the case with pure cysts. I decline to biopsy nodules when the ultrasound reveals a very smooth and clearly visible border, a thin, dark rim called a halo all the way around it. I also will not biopsy if there is an absence of calcification inside the nodule (an "eggshell" calcification around the nodule is actually a good sign) and no increased blood flow. Such a nodule can be observed even if it is only a little bigger than 1 centimeter. I will hold off on performing an FNA if it is 15 millimeters or smaller.

If I decide that an FNA biopsy is necessary but can't see the nodule because it is deep under the skin, I will want to use ultrasound guidance with the FNA. This way, I can be sure I suck up nodule tissue, not something else.

If the FNA biopsy indicates that the nodule is either cancerous or suspicious for cancer, or if it shows follicular neoplasm, the patient must have surgery. In cases of cancer, the whole thyroid must be removed as soon as possible.

With follicular neoplasm and nodules that are suspicious for cancer, only the part of the thyroid containing the nodule is removed (a partial thyroidectomy). While the patient is still on the operating table, a pathologist will examine the excised nodule under a microscope. If the nodule is cancerous, the rest of the thyroid is immediately removed. If the nodule is benign, the surgery is completed. As discussed earlier, a patient can live quite normally with only a partial thyroid, provided that it is a healthy thyroid.

Pathologic exams done during an operation are not as reliable as those carried out after appropriate preparation and staining of the tissue, which is done postoperatively. Occasionally, the intraoperative diagnosis is overturned by a follow-up pathologic study. In this case, the patient must undergo another surgery if the diagnosis turns out to show cancer.

FNA Flaws. Although FNA is an excellent test, it is not perfect. It has been reported that FNA diagnosis finds 95 percent of thyroid cancers. This means it misses 5 percent of them.

If the FNA biopsy indicates the nodule is benign, but the nodule is growing, I believe it should be cut out and examined. Though surgery is invasive, the risks are too great to allow an actively growing nodule to remain in the thyroid. Too frequently these types of nodules turn out to be malignant.

Another 5 percent of FNA biopsies are classified as nondiagnostic. Either not enough tissue was removed from the nodule for a diagnosis, or the sample was not preserved properly.

If the biopsy is nondiagnostic, the procedure will need to be repeated. If the FNA is nondiagnostic the second time, I will not repeat the test a third time. I monitor the nodule with ultrasound in 3 months, then 6 months after that, and 12 months after that to see if it has grown.

If the nodule hasn't grown after this time, it will most likely never grow, so clinical examination of the thyroid (an examination by touching) should be sufficient. But if I ever suspect that the nodule has grown, I perform a new thyroid ultrasound at once.

Shrinking a Nodule. If a nodule is not hot and is not growing but is of cosmetic concern, patients may want it shrunk. Currently, there are two methods used in the U.S. to shrink nodules.

One way to shrink a nodule is by giving patients thyroid hormone. Ingesting thyroid hormone (Synthroid, for example) increases hormone levels in the blood, which triggers the pituitary to cut back production of TSH. Since TSH stimulates the growth of thyroid tissue, curtailing its production should shrink thyroid tissue and thyroid nodules.

Unfortunately, there is no conclusive evidence that cutting TSH production shrinks nodules consistently (it has a chance to work if TSH is elevated at the start). Furthermore, there are risks associated with giving healthy people thyroid hormone. Finally, about 30 percent of all nodules shrink on their own.

The second method for shrinking nodules, alcohol ablation, is more reliable. In this therapy, ethyl alcohol is injected into the nodule to shrink the tissue by killing it. Some patients need multiple injections given at two-month intervals. But for the majority, one injection is sufficient. With alcohol ablation of cold nodules, there is no risk of inducing hyperthyroidism as there is with giving thyroid hormones. If the nodule is hot, the patient should be treated with antithyroid medications for four to eight weeks prior to alcohol injection to avoid any hyperthyroidism after injection.

The needle and syringe used for alcohol ablation are the same size as those used for FNA, and the procedure is likewise performed with ultrasound guidance. Typically, the physician injects 1 to 2 cubic centimeters of alcohol, which can be seen spreading through the nodule via ultrasound.

Most patients experience only mild discomfort during the procedure, although some people (about 10 percent) feel a relatively intense burning pain after the injection. This pain usually lasts only a couple of minutes.

New Treatments. Two new methods of shrinking nodules have been developed and administered with success in Italy and France. Italian doctors have begun successfully shrinking benign nodules with laser ablation. They place a needle into the nodule (as in the FNA and alcohol-injection procedures), then thread a fiber-optic filament through the needle into the nodule. One to four filaments are temporarily planted inside the nodule. Then a laser is fired at the filaments to heat the nodule tissue and kill it. Afterward, the filaments are removed. It takes several weeks for the nodule to shrink.

The French have designed a machine that focuses ultrasound energy into a single beam. At the same time, the machine images

> # Red Flag
>
> If you are planning to have any ablation (shrinking) treatment, ask your doctor if he or she has checked that the nodule is benign and has not grown.

the thyroid, enabling the doctor to target the energy precisely on the nodule. When fired, this focused ultrasound beam heats up the nodule tissue, causing its cells to die and the nodule to shrink.

Both of these methods are more expensive, more cumbersome, and currently have no better success than alcohol injections.

What Makes Doctors Typically Decide to Operate on Nodules?

Nodules should be removed surgically if they are large, malignant, suspicious for cancer, growing, or causing symptoms from pressure.

Goiters

A goiter is an enlarged thyroid gland. Goiters vary greatly in size. Some are detectable only by touch; others make patients look as if they've swallowed a softball. In iodine-deficient parts of the world, goiters can be as large as cantaloupes. Most goiters are all contained in the neck area, but some will spread downward and behind the breastbone, or sternum, into the chest cavity. Such goiters are called substernal goiters.

There are many causes of goiters, not all of which are understood. In some cases, a goiter is part of another thyroid disorder and doesn't need any specific treatment but resolves with the thyroid condition or disappears spontaneously over time.

Having a goiter doesn't automatically mean you have an underactive or overactive thyroid. The thyroids of most patients with goiters function normally.

What Are the Symptoms of Goiter?

Most goiters give no symptoms to the patient, but sometimes large goiters, substernal goiters, or goiters containing thyroid cancer may cause the following symptoms:

- Hoarseness
- Difficulty swallowing or breathing
- Chronic cough
- Tightness in the throat
- Discomfort inside the goiter

Sometimes multinodular goiters present mechanical problems, such as impeded breathing or swallowing. I typically ask people to raise their arms in my office during examinations. Some people with substernal goiters have difficulty breathing only when they raise their arms to comb their hair or brush their teeth. The collarbones and ribs lift with their arms, causing the thoracic outlet (the upper opening of the thoracic cage) to push upward against the goiter, exerting pressure. If someone has a significant substernal goiter, within one minute, he or she will grow red in the face, have difficulty breathing, and see the veins in the neck engorge. This reaction is known as Pemberton's sign.

How Many Different Types of Goiters Are There?

There are three major types of goiters.

Goiter and Graves' Disease. Most patients with Graves' disease have some accompanying thyroid enlargement. Usually, these goiters are palpable, but they are not always visible. Goiters associated with Graves' disease rarely present mechanical problems, such as difficulty in swallowing or breathing. The enlargement is uniform and is called diffuse goiter. When touched, the Graves' goiter is softer than a normal healthy thyroid. There are no accompanying nodules. Putting the stethoscope over the Graves' goiter will sometimes allow the physician to hear a murmur of blood flowing through the gland— this is called thyroid bruit. When treated with radioactive iodine, the goiter shrinks completely.

Goiter and Hashimoto's Thyroiditis. In the early stages of Hashimoto's, some patients develop uniform thyroid enlargement or diffuse goiter because of the influx of lymphocytes (immune cells that cause inflammation), which triggers swelling of the gland. Rarely, the thyroid may swell to three or four times larger than normal. However, these goiters eventually shrink as the inflammation destroys the thyroid. They virtually never cause problems with breathing or swallowing.

But when the inflammation is most intense, the patient may experience mild tenderness in the throat. A man might notice this when he puts on a tie. With Hashimoto's associated goiters, we treat the patient for hypothyroidism, not for goiter.

Multinodular Goiters. Historically, most goiters have been caused by iodine deficiency. In the U.S., this type of goiter has virtually disappeared since the mandatory introduction of iodized salt, which ensures that our population gets adequate amounts of iodine.

Most commonly in this country, we see multinodular goiters. They look like iodine-deficiency goiters, but they are rarely as large and are usually lumpy, as if someone tucked a bunch of grapes just under the skin.

We don't know why they develop, although there are many theories. One possible cause is the presence of goitrogens, such as soybeans. Goitrogens are substances in the environment, including food, that prevent the thyroid from absorbing iodine. If iodine absorption is inhibited, the pituitary boosts TSH production, which stimulates the thyroid to grow, causing a goiter. This is only a theory because in most cases, no connection between diet and goiter can be established.

Goiters also run in families, but not necessarily for genetic reasons. The case may be that families tend to eat the same foods or simply that they share a common environment. We know what multinodular goiters are, but we don't know why they form.

We do know that elderly people are more prone to multinodular goiters than the young are. Often, we find older people who have them also have slightly suppressed TSH (just a little lower than normal) but no symptoms of hyperthyroidism. This indicates that some of the nodules are losing their dependence on TSH for regulation. When these individuals receive large amounts of iodine—as with the contrast from a CT scan or the drug amiodarone—they may develop full-blown hyperthyroidism that lasts for several months—until the iodine is spent.

Frequently, you can see the multinodular goiters, but many elderly people reject surgery or radioactive iodine to shrink the goiter if it is merely for cosmetic reasons. In these cases, no treatment is necessary. Most multinodular goiters are not overtly toxic, although some may have slight abnormalities upon examination in the lab.

How Are Goiters Evaluated?

Ultrasound is an excellent tool to assess multinodular goiters that are limited to the neck, as most are. Unfortunately, it is not useful for trying to evaluate and measure substernal parts of a goiter because ultrasound can't penetrate bone.

The best way to evaluate a substernal goiter is with a non-contrast CT scan. Again, the iodine in contrast CT scans can cause hyperthyroidism by feeding and transforming borderline-toxic nodules into toxic ones.

Sometimes physicians want to see the patient's blood vessels. Normally, a contrast CT is used for this purpose because it provides clear delineation of the vessels. But in the case of goiters, we need to administer an MRI instead.

Both the MRI and CT scans not only show the goiter's size, but they also reveal whether it is pressing on the windpipe or other structures in the chest cavity. This enables us to determine the best treatment for each individual.

A radioactive iodine uptake and scan provide similar information about the size and activity of thyroid tissue, but these evaluations can be misleading because parts of a multinodular goiter may absorb iodine poorly. Therefore, these tests are not used to evaluate size and shape of multinodular goiters. However, if we are interested in function within the goiter, this is the way to go.

If the imaging by ultrasound, MRI, or CT reveals a dominant nodule in the goiter—one that stands out as larger than the others—it should be evaluated further with an FNA. It could be cancerous. The risk of cancer in a multinodular goiter is probably a little less than when only one nodule is present.

How Are Goiters Treated?

Most patients with thyroid enlargements exhibit no symptoms, and many have no cosmetic concerns. I don't believe such people need any particular treatment except for being monitored periodically to ensure that there is no further growth. Since goiters that grow do so very slowly, the checkups need to be continued indefinitely.

A patient with a goiter should be treated if the goiter is:

- Causing mechanical problems (breathing, swallowing)
- Substernal, even if there are no mechanical symptoms (with some exceptions)
- Unsightly

- Growing
- Suspicious for cancer

Surgical Removal. The primary treatment option for multinodular goiter is surgery. Decisions about surgery are made on an individual basis. I frequently monitor unhealthy elderly patients with substernal goiters who have no accompanying symptoms, especially if they have lung or heart problems that would make surgery risky.

After surgery, the patient ends up with a scar, which can be a disappointment if he or she wanted a goiter removed to improve cosmetic appearance. However, the scar is only 1 to 1½ inches long. Twenty years ago, the incision would have looked like a smiley face drawn from one side of the neck to the other.

Most goiters can be removed with a neck incision, but some large, substernal goiters require opening the chest with a thoracotomy and sawing through the bone. This type of operation requires the assistance of a cardiothoracic surgeon (a specialist who does such surgeries on a regular basis).

Of course, this is a major surgery and carries much more risk than a simple neck incision. Also, the patient will have a more conspicuous scar.

But in many cases, the surgical approach depends on the skill of the surgeon. More skillful surgeons are less invasive and more often go in through the neck.

Patients need to be carefully prepared for surgery. Some will have suppressed TSH and mild hyperthyroidism; others will suffer from real hyperthyroidism. These patients should take antithyroid medications for several weeks prior to surgery to normalize the thyroid. To avoid any surprises during surgery, the vocal cords and any windpipe constriction should be examined in advance.

The surgeon decides how much of the goiter to remove on a case-by-case basis. But because the goiter could return, surgeons usually take out as much thyroid tissue as possible without creating unnecessary risks to the voice box nerves and the parathyroid glands.

Postoperative complications and recovery rate are the same as after surgery for thyroid cancer, described in detail in chapter 8.

After a surgery that removes most of the thyroid, thyroid hormone replacement therapy is necessary to counter postoperative hypothyroidism. Some studies suggest that thyroid hormone replacement therapy prevents regrowth of the goiter when a significant amount of thyroid tissue remains after surgery.

Thyroid Hormone Pills. Thyroid hormone pills can be used as an alternative to surgery. They gradually decrease goiter size in about two-thirds of patients.

However, the shrinking is slow (from two to three months) and is usually insufficient to relieve symptoms of compression (if any). Also, individuals with overactive thyroids will not benefit from ingesting more thyroid hormone. However, hormone therapy is worth trying if the patient's TSH is on the high side of normal and there are no symptoms.

Radioactive Iodine. Radioactive iodine is another treatment option. The doses used are generally between 30 and 100 millicuries. Between half and two-thirds of patients experience shrinking of the goiter over a six-month period.

Most of the data gathered on this form of treatment comes from Europe and shows that nearly all patients eventually have some benefit. The greatest amount of shrinking occurs within the first several weeks, but the process may continue for more than a year. About 3 percent of the patients have some thyroid pain after treatment, but almost no one requires surgery.

One problem with radioactive iodine treatment is that there are legal limits as to how much radioactivity a physician can administer to the individual with an intact thyroid before the patient becomes a public risk and must be hospitalized; 30 millicuries is the limit for office treatment. However, sometimes that amount is not strong enough to shrink the goiter because large goiters do not take up all the iodine given. In such cases, the doctor may have to deliver the radioactive iodine several times on subsequent visits or administer a higher dose while the patient is hospitalized.

Iodine uptake can be improved by giving the patient an injection of artificial (recombinant) human TSH before delivering the radiation. This synthetic TSH recently became available and is used to help manage patients with thyroid cancer.

Increasing the TSH level artificially stimulates the thyroid to work harder and extract more iodine from the blood. Afterward, when radioactive iodine is administered, there is much greater absorption into the goiter. Studies show that the amount of absorption approximately doubles. In this case, one dose of 30 millicuries is usually sufficient to shrink the goiter. Unfortunately, artificial TSH is expensive, and insurance companies will not pay for it because this therapy has not yet been approved by the FDA.

Large, substernal goiters should not be treated with radioactive iodine because the iodine may cause the goiter to swell before it begins shrinking. We can't risk any swelling in the chest; therefore, large substernal goiters must be treated with surgery.

Another reason for preferring surgery to radioactive iodine therapy is that cancer may be hidden in the substernal portion of the goiter, where it cannot be biopsied and discovered prior to treatment.

In the future, as more data is gathered on the outcomes of radioactive iodine treatment, people with substernal goiters may also become candidates for radioactive iodine therapy.

Although not as common as hypothyroidism and hyperthyroidism, dealing with thyroid nodules and multinodular goiters makes up a significant portion of my work. Most of the time these are benign conditions not requiring treatment, but they always need careful evaluation and follow-up.

Chapter 8

Thyroid Cancers

T hyroid cancer is the most common cancer of the endocrine glands (pituitary, adrenals, ovaries, testicles, pancreas, and parathyroid glands). In recent years, the incidence of most cancers has fallen, but thyroid cancers have risen. About 30,000 new cases of thyroid cancer were reported in the United States in 2006. Roughly 21,000 of these were women; 9,000 were men. Approximately 1,500 people died of thyroid cancer in 2005: 850 women and 650 men.

Diagnosis in the Early Stages

Many patients, especially in the early stages of thyroid cancer, do not have any symptoms. However, as the cancer develops, symptoms may include a lump or nodule in the front of the neck, hoarseness or difficulty speaking, swollen lymph nodes, difficulty swallowing or breathing, and pain in the throat. Most thyroid cancers are diagnosed in the early stages of the disease as visible or palpable nodules. In fact, most of the increase in the number of newly diagnosed thyroid cancers consists of the small, early cases. About 49 percent of the increase is comprised of cancers smaller than

10 millimeters, and 87 percent are cancers smaller than 20 millimeters. Thankfully, this suggests that the increase in the incidence of thyroid cancers is because we are now better at diagnosing small, early cancers, using the new imaging technologies—not because of a real increase in the number of new cancers.

Are There Different Types of Malignant Thyroid Tumors?

There are two major categories of malignant, or cancerous, thyroid tumors. The various types of thyroid cancers are grouped accordingly.

Well Differentiated. Papillary and follicular thyroid carcinomas account for 80 to 90 percent of all thyroid cancers. These cancers develop from follicular thyroid cells, the ones that produce T4.

They are classified as well-differentiated thyroid cancers, meaning their cells have a very similar size and shape. A pathologist can readily recognize this type of cancer and its origin. These cancers are well behaved, as far as cancers go, and relatively easy to manage. They grow more slowly than other cancers and are less likely to be fatal.

The treatment and management of these cancers are similar. If detected early, most papillary and follicular thyroid cancer can be treated successfully.

Poorly Differentiated. Poorly differentiated thyroid cancers have a jumbled appearance. Pathologists have a difficult time identifying poorly differentiated cancers and cannot determine their point of origin.

Anaplastic thyroid carcinoma is the least common and accounts for only 1 to 2 percent of all thyroid cancer. This cancer is very difficult to control and treat because it is extremely aggressive.

Medullary thyroid carcinoma accounts for 5 to 10 percent of all thyroid cancers. It begins in parts of the thyroid called C cells, which have nothing to do with controlling the metabolism but play a small role in calcium metabolism. Medullary cancer is either sporadic (occurring randomly in different individuals) or familial (running in families with certain genetic mutations). Genetic testing is very important in the management of these cancers.

When medullary cancer is confined to the thyroid gland, survival rates at ten years after diagnosis are around 90 percent. If the cancer has spread to lymph nodes in the neck, the rate is 70 percent. If it has metastasized further, the survival rate drops to about 20 percent. Medullary cancer is much easier to treat and control if it is found before it spreads to other parts of the body.

Other Malignancies Seen in the Thyroid. Thyroid lymphoma is a malignancy that arises from immune cells (lymphocytes). It is a rare disease that occurs 75 times more often in individuals who have Hashimoto's thyroiditis than in the rest of the population.

Well-Differentiated Thyroid Cancers

The well-differentiated papillary and follicular thyroid cancers make up the vast majority of cases. These are the cancers that we describe to patients as the best kind of cancer one can have. Most of the time, we can cure these cancers using surgery and radioactive iodine.

The Most Common: Papillary Cancer

Papillary carcinoma, also known as papillary adenocarcinoma, makes up 70 percent of all thyroid cancers. It usually grows as a solitary lump or mass in one wing of the thyroid. The disease is most prevalent in women between ages 30 and 50. There are about 20,000 new cases of papillary cancer annually and about 1,200 deaths every year.

Papillary cancer grows slowly, usually does not have a shell or capsule around it, and frequently spreads to the nearby lymph nodes in the neck. In 40 to 50 percent of patients, the cancer has spread to the lymph nodes at the time of diagnosis. Probably as many as 80 percent have microscopic spread. But this does not exacerbate the condition; most of the time, it can be cured.

If papillary cancer is not caught early, however, it can travel to other parts of the body, especially the lungs and the bones. This has occurred in about 10 percent of patients at the time of diagnosis. At this point, the cancer is much more dangerous but still treatable and curable with surgery, radioactive iodine-131, external radiation, or other methods.

Almost all stage 1, well-differentiated thyroid cancers can be cured. But when the malignancy has spread outside the neck, it is harder to cure. Nonetheless, only about 6 percent of all papillary cancer patients will eventually die of the condition.

The prognosis for survival depends on certain features of the cancer, including size, the degree of metastasis, and the patient's age. The larger the tumor at the time of diagnosis, the worse the prognosis. Cancers that are less than 2 centimeters—1 inch equals 2.54 centimeters—are categorized as small. Average-sized tumors are between 2 and 4 centimeters. Anything bigger than 4 centimeters is considered to be a large tumor. Studies suggest that about 50 percent of patients will survive an additional 20 years even if the cancer is larger than 7 centimeters (a little less than 3 inches in diameter) when it is diagnosed.

For well-differentiated thyroid cancers (both papillary and follicular) that are less than 2 centimeters, the cure rate approaches 100 percent. These statistics underscore the importance of catching the disease and treating it early.

If the cancer spreads from the thyroid gland into the surrounding tissue (the windpipe, esophagus, and so on), the prognosis is worse—the risk of death increases fivefold. Of course, those with distant metastases at diagnosis have the worst prognosis.

Subtypes of Papillary Cancer

When well-differentiated thyroid cancers are examined under the microscope, sometimes the cells do not look exactly typical or clumps of cells form atypical shapes. Depending on these atypical features, a pathologist will classify the cancer as one of the variants.

All the variants of papillary thyroid cancer are more aggressive than papillary thyroid cancer itself and have slightly worse prognoses. The follicular variant is the most common subtype, accounting for about 10 percent of all papillary cancers. The tall cell variant represents about 1 percent. The other forms are even rarer. The variants include:

- Follicular variant
- Insular variant
- Tall cell variant
- Hurtle cell variant
- Columnar variant
- Diffuse sclerosing variant
- Clear cell variant
- Trabecular variant

Unlike most other cancers, the age of the patient plays a role too. If you are between 20 and 45 years of age, your prognosis is better than if you are younger or older. Also, men fare slightly worse than women, no matter what their age.

Follicular Cancer: An Excellent Prognosis

Follicular carcinoma (follicular adenocarcinoma) is the second most common type of thyroid cancer, representing about 10 percent of all thyroid cancers. Slightly more aggressive than papillary cancer, it tends to spread through the bloodstream within the thyroid and then invade other organs, most often the lungs and bones.

Like papillary cancer, follicular cancer has an excellent prognosis and can be cured with surgery and radioactive iodine. The prognosis is worse when the tumor spreads beyond the thyroid to other locations in the body.

Follicular cancer cells are so well differentiated that pathologists frequently can't tell, in looking at cells obtained by FNA, whether the tumor is malignant or benign.

Sometimes the pathologist can distinguish between benign and malignant follicular nodules, but frequently doctors send patients to surgery without knowing. During the surgery, the pathologist determines whether the tumor is malignant or benign by examining a frozen sample of tumor tissue.

If the nodule is benign, the surgeon will remove only the part of the thyroid that contains the tumor. If the nodule is malignant, the surgeon will remove the entire thyroid.

What Are the Doctors Looking for Under the Microscope?

Cells in the body constantly divide to replace the older ones that die. During the division, the cells must make duplicates of all the genes contained in them. During this duplication, occasional errors occur. These errors are called mutations. Most of these errors are repaired quickly; if the error cannot be repaired, the cell is destroyed and absorbed. Some of these cells would become cancers if not removed. Luckily, most malignant cells are swept from the body by our very alert immune systems. But when a malignant cell evades detection by the immune system, it grows into cancer.

As far as we know, every cancer begins from just one aberrant cell. All cancer cells are the offspring or clones of that one cell that managed to evade the immune system. We call this a monoclonal origin.

To be cancerous, a cell must have three features. It must have the ability to:

- Divide endlessly
- Invade the surrounding tissue
- Spread (metastasize)

Invading the surrounding tissue means the malignant tumor grows directly into neighboring tissue like a spreading blob. In contrast, when benign tumors grow, they simply nudge or push aside neighboring tissue; they don't infiltrate it.

To metastasize means to spread anywhere in the body through the lymphatic or blood circulatory system. Though cancer can theoretically spread anywhere, each cancer has a propensity to travel to certain locations.

Both follicular cancer and benign follicular adenoma nodules are contained within a capsule, which is filled with small nests of thyroid cells. To distinguish between follicular cancer and benign follicular adenoma, pathologists look to see whether the tumor has broken out of the capsule and whether thyroid cells have spilled out of the nests and invaded the blood vessels. If they observe either of these events, they will classify the tumor as cancerous.

Who Gets Thyroid Cancer—and Why?

Many times patients ask me, "Why did I get this disease? Is it my diet that did it or something else?"

Unfortunately, there is nothing one can do to avoid thyroid cancer altogether. The causes of both papillary and follicular cancer are largely unknown, but we are aware of several things that contribute to a higher risk:

- A family history of these cancers

- Having had radiation treatment of the head and neck

- Having lived near Chernobyl, the site of the worst nuclear reactor accident in history, or the Marshall Islands in the Pacific Ocean, which were unexpectedly exposed to fallout during nuclear testing

- Individuals with certain genetic syndromes, such as Cowden syndrome, Gardner syndrome, and familial adenomatous polyposis

People in these risk groups should be examined for nodules on a regular basis.

Generally, papillary cancer is more prevalent in women than in men. It occurs most frequently in people under 50 but is more aggressive in elderly people.

How Do Doctors Detect Well-Differentiated Thyroid Cancer?

Thyroid cancer begins as a thyroid nodule and is diagnosed in the same way as benign nodules (see chapter 7).

Regina

Regina, 52, felt a lump in her throat while putting on makeup. She called my office immediately, and we made an appointment for the same week.

When I examined her neck, I found that the lump was rock-hard, which suggested it wasn't an ordinary nodule. Upon measuring it with an ultrasound, I discovered it was average size for an ordinary thyroid nodule: 20 millimeters by 15 millimeters by 15 millimeters (about the size of a grape). This was a good sign.

But the ultrasound revealed something else. The nodule was splotched with grainy areas of calcification—an indication of possible thyroid cancer. I followed up with a fine needle aspiration biopsy. Regina's results came back positive. She had papillary thyroid cancer. But she had no symptoms other than the lump and felt perfectly healthy. Most of the time, patients with thyroid cancer will not have any symptoms. Thyroid function is also normal in a vast majority of the patients. Because of that, periodic examinations of the neck are necessary. We cannot expect to discover thyroid cancer at an early stage by waiting for symptoms. Regina's cancer grew in the area close to the skin and was discovered while still small.

I immediately scheduled Regina for surgery.

Regina's surgery took place on a Thursday morning, three weeks after the cancer was diagnosed. The surgeon removed her thyroid completely, along with those lymph nodes nearest the thyroid that appeared enlarged so that they could be examined by a pathologist for any spread of the cancer. She went home Friday afternoon and returned to work on Monday. It appeared that all the cancer had been cut out.

I saw Regina again a week later. The only sign of the surgery was a small scar on her neck, a little more than an inch long. She hid it by buttoning her shirt collar to the top. Since Regina's thyroid had to be completely removed, she was hypothyroid and had to take 100 micrograms of T4 a day (she would have to take supplements for the rest of her life, but this was a small price to pay for beating cancer). In addition, I prescribed 1,000 milligrams of calcium per day and 1000 international units of vitamin D per day. I often do this to ensure blood calcium levels stay normal in patients whose parathyroid glands (which control calcium) are accidentally removed or damaged during thyroid surgery.

During our follow-up visit, I shared Regina's pathology report with her. (A pathology report details specifics about the cancer that the pathologist has discovered in the tissue and cells when they are examined under a microscope.) The surgeon had found a small, 15-millimeter papillary thyroid cancer in the right wing of her thyroid, as we expected. When I explained that the cancer had spread to multiple lymph nodes in her neck, tears streamed down her cheeks. But I calmed Regina, explaining that this is quite common with papillary cancer and that the surgeon had already removed these cancerous lymph nodes.

Once cancer metastasizes to the lymph nodes, people panic and often fear the worst. But papillary thyroid cancer is different from other cancers. Even when it spreads into the neighboring lymph nodes, it is still very curable.

Then I told her that what we call her surgical margins were not affected by the cancer. "This means that all of your cancer is contained in the tissue we removed. That's great news," I explained. "There is no sign of any cancer remnants left in your neck." Obviously, she was very pleased to hear this.

I advised Regina, as I advise all my patients, to keep a copy of her pathology report because sometimes the cancer returns 15 to 20 years after the first surgery. If that should happen, this original report would help her doctor know how best to treat her.

To many, the word *cancer* means imminent death. But most thyroid cancers grow slowly and can be completely cured with adequate therapy. At her next appointment, Regina was optimistic about her future. She had read a great deal about papillary cancer and was reassured by her treatment and our follow-up plans.

A few months later, as is customary, I decided to use radioactive iodine to ensure that all the cancer cells were gone. Regina had some uptake in the neck after the tracer dose. The scan was done 24 hours after she swallowed a capsule containing 2 millicuries of I-123. We expected to find uptake in the neck because a surgeon can rarely remove every last trace of thyroid tissue from the neck. We followed up the scan with radioactive iodine ablation, using

100 millicuries of I-131, which appeared to have destroyed all the cancer. She now takes 125 micrograms of levothyroxin daily, which is slightly higher than the dose she would need to manage if she just had hypothyroidism.

Regina returns for checkups every six months to make sure the cancer hasn't returned. She now expects to see her children grow up—and her grandchildren too!

Staging Well-Differentiated Thyroid Cancer

After surgery and radioactive iodine tests and scans, a physician will have all the information needed to stage a disease. Regina, for example, had stage 1 papillary cancer.

How and Why Do We Stage a Patient's Cancer?

The purpose of staging thyroid cancer is to classify patients according to the degree of severity of their cancer: stage 1, 2, 3, or 4. The lower the stage, the better the prognosis. Staging is one of the tools that help physicians select an appropriate therapy and follow-up regimes for each patient.

There are several staging systems, which means none of them is perfect. These systems were developed by various institutions. The Mayo Clinic developed two staging systems, and Ohio State University developed one. Also, there is an international staging system called TNM, which can be used to classify all types of cancers based on tumor size (T), lymph node (N) involvement, and presence or absence of metastasis (M). This classification works well for most cancers and is useful for thyroid cancer too.

With thyroid cancers, however, the patient's age has a prognostic value, and the TNM now includes an age factor in the classification. Prior TNM systems did not use age because age is not clinically important in other cancers. I prefer the latest system developed at the Mayo Clinic, MACIS, because I think it better fits the clinical features of thyroid cancers. This system assigns a score (number) to class the severity of the cancer.

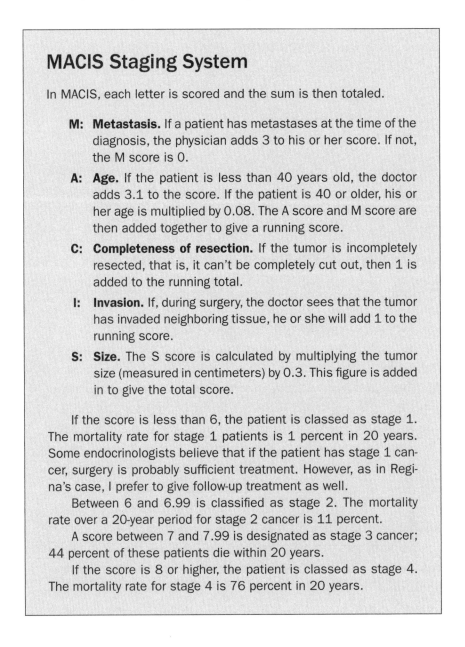

MACIS Staging System

In MACIS, each letter is scored and the sum is then totaled.

M: **Metastasis.** If a patient has metastases at the time of the diagnosis, the physician adds 3 to his or her score. If not, the M score is 0.

A: **Age.** If the patient is less than 40 years old, the doctor adds 3.1 to the score. If the patient is 40 or older, his or her age is multiplied by 0.08. The A score and M score are then added together to give a running score.

C: **Completeness of resection.** If the tumor is incompletely resected, that is, it can't be completely cut out, then 1 is added to the running total.

I: **Invasion.** If, during surgery, the doctor sees that the tumor has invaded neighboring tissue, he or she will add 1 to the running score.

S: **Size.** The S score is calculated by multiplying the tumor size (measured in centimeters) by 0.3. This figure is added in to give the total score.

If the score is less than 6, the patient is classed as stage 1. The mortality rate for stage 1 patients is 1 percent in 20 years. Some endocrinologists believe that if the patient has stage 1 cancer, surgery is probably sufficient treatment. However, as in Regina's case, I prefer to give follow-up treatment as well.

Between 6 and 6.99 is classified as stage 2. The mortality rate over a 20-year period for stage 2 cancer is 11 percent.

A score between 7 and 7.99 is designated as stage 3 cancer; 44 percent of these patients die within 20 years.

If the score is 8 or higher, the patient is classed as stage 4. The mortality rate for stage 4 is 76 percent in 20 years.

Surgical Treatment for Well-Differentiated Thyroid Cancer

Once thyroid cancer is diagnosed, it has to be surgically removed. How much of the thyroid gland should be cut out for small, well-differentiated cancers (1 centimeter and smaller) is a topic of debate.

Partial versus Total Thyroidectomy

Generally speaking, if small papillary or follicular tumors are confined to one lobe and there is no lymph node involvement or spreading beyond the thyroid, the tumors can be treated by removing just the part of the thyroid that contains the nodule. This is called a partial thyroidectomy or a lobectomy if only one lobe is removed.

In such cases, the patient won't become hypothyroid after surgery. Even half of the thyroid can manufacture enough thyroid hormone to maintain normal hormone levels in the blood.

However, a few endocrinologists think that all thyroid cancers require a total thyroidectomy. A total or near-total thyroidectomy is customary for larger cancers (larger than 1 centimeter) or even small tumors if the patient has a history of radiation treatment. (Since radiation-induced cancers are frequently present on several sites inside the thyroid, only complete removal of the entire gland guarantees removal of all the cancerous tissue.)

A total thyroidectomy can be involved and requires great surgical skill. The typical operation lasts three and a half to four hours, although some of my patients have had surgeries that lasted up to eight hours!

Among other painstaking tasks, the surgeon must gently separate thyroid tissue from small but important structures, such as nerves and blood vessels, before removing the thyroid. These structures are so important that the surgeon will preserve them, even if that means leaving a trace of thyroid tissue on them. Because of this, total thyroidectomies are rarely 100 percent successful in removing all traces of thyroid tissue.

Subtotal Thyroidectomy

In a subtotal thyroidectomy, the surgeon intentionally leaves a few more thyroid remnants in place to minimize the risk of injuring the nearby voice box nerve. These tissue remnants are located in the back of the thyroid near the voice box.

It is critical that the surgeon examine the lymph nodes in the areas of the neck that drain the thyroid gland. Every lymph node that is suspicious for cancer—hard, round, and enlarged—should be removed during surgery and examined under the microscope by the pathologist to see whether it is cancerous.

If the nodes closest to the thyroid are clean, there is no need for the surgeon to look further. These are always the first to be invaded by papillary cancer. (Follicular cancer is most commonly metastasized by the bloodstream.)

Complications of Thyroidectomy

A thyroidectomy usually does not require the surgeon to open any major body cavity, and blood transfusions are not needed. Thyroidectomies are much less risky than, for example, open-heart surgery. Nonetheless, cutting into the neck can cause some collateral damage, such as severing the vocal cord nerves or destroying the parathyroid glands.

One study of 5,583 thyroid surgeries found that 1.3 percent of the patients had permanent damage to one of their vocal nerves. These patients became permanently hoarse.

Cutting both the vocal nerves is an extremely rare complication that endangers the patient's life. When the vocal nerves are both cut, the vocal cords snap shut, causing labored breathing (stridor).

New Data Every Day

It is important to note that new data about thyroid cancer accumulates every day; therefore, current recommendations may change. I think that even somewhat larger cancers can be cured effectively by surgery alone, provided there is no metastasis.

Sometimes, the surgeon must puncture the trachea to enable the patient to get air.

Another complication is hypocalcemia, caused by slicing some or all four of the nearby parathyroid glands. If this happens, the calcium levels in the blood drop to abnormally low levels within 24 hours of surgery.

Hypocalcemia occurs in about 10 percent of total thyroidectomy cases and is usually transient. It is easily corrected with calcium and vitamin D supplements.

However, accidentally removing all four parathyroid glands induces permanent hypoparathyroidism, which causes low calcium and high phosphorus levels in the blood. Fortunately, treatment with calcium and vitamin D usually normalizes these levels. But these patients will have to take supplements permanently.

All other complications, such as infection and bleeding, are rare and are treated as in other types of surgery. Frequently, there will be some numbness around the surgical scar, like around any other scar caused by a deep cut.

Additional Treatment for Well-Differentiated Thyroid Cancer

Some doctors still feel that all patients should have follow-up therapy, but generally speaking, further treatment is unnecessary after surgery if the tumor is small and hasn't spread to the lymph nodes. But additional therapy *is* necessary if the tumor is large or the cancer has spread to the lymph nodes, as in Regina's case.

Radioactive Iodine Therapy

The next step in such cases is for the patient to have radioactive iodine therapy, also called ablation, to kill any remaining cancer cells as well as any remaining healthy thyroid tissue. This treatment also enables the physician to determine the final staging of the cancer (see page 141) because it either reveals or rules out metastases.

The patient swallows radioactive iodine in a capsule. The iodine is taken up by the thyroid gland, and the dose of radiation coming from the iodine is enough to destroy the cancerous and normal thyroid cells but not high enough to damage other normal tissues. This is done on an outpatient basis for most patients.

Radioactive iodine therapy is generally done about six to eight weeks after surgery. This avoids normal postoperative swelling, which would impede the free flow of blood necessary to deliver the iodine to the cells. In ordinary circumstances, treatment should not be delayed for more than three months following the thyroidectomy.

Preparing for Radioactive Iodine Therapy. Since thyroid cancer cells are never as good at picking up iodine as normal thyroid tissue, we create conditions prior to the ablation to maximize absorption by the cancer. This is achieved in two ways. One is to increase the TSH level over the 25 microunits per milliliter, which will stimulate any thyroid cell to work hard and pick up the iodine. The second is to deplete the body of iodine so there is nothing to compete with radioactive iodine once it is administered.

Increasing TSH to the level higher than 25 microunits per milliliter can be achieved in two different ways.

The first involves taking patients off thyroid hormones (T4) five weeks prior to their radioactive iodine treatment. One week after their T4 is stopped, we give 25 micrograms of T3 per day for two weeks to minimize the length of time they will have symptoms of hypothyroidism.

Then patients take no hormones for two weeks before treatment. This causes their TSH levels to increase. We want the TSH level high to stimulate all the remaining cells—thyroid and thyroid cancer cells—to absorb the radioactive iodine when it is given.

It takes five weeks for the TSH to climb to 25 in all patients, which is the minimum level needed to stimulate significant pickup by the cancer cells. Most of the patients' TSH is much higher than 25 by the time of treatment.

The second way to increase the TSH level involves the use of synthetic human recombinant TSH. In 2006, the FDA approved the use of synthetic human recombinant TSH in low-risk patients for this purpose. Low-risk patients are those who have stage 1 disease. We administer 0.9 milligrams of human recombinant TSH by injection into the muscle on two consecutive days. This is enough to raise the TSH level in the blood much higher than the 25 necessary for treatment. Treatment is administered about 24 hours after the second injection. This approach is more expensive, but it prevents the patient being hypothyroid.

To minimize the body iodine load, we put patients on a low-iodine diet for two weeks prior to their treatment to deplete their bodies of iodine. This way, when the radioactive iodine is given, there is no competition. To help patients stick to this diet, we provide them with a low-iodine cookbook, published by the Thyroid Cancer Survivors' Association, Inc., also available on the organization's website, *www.thyca.org*. Some doctors keep patients on a longer diet, up to four weeks.

When a patient is taken off of thyroid medication in preparation for treatment, during the final two weeks before radioactive iodine treatment, the patients are all profoundly hypothyroid. In addition, low-iodine diets are notoriously bland, and many people complain about them and have food cravings. Most patients feel tired and have to push themselves to carry out routine tasks. A few patients feel fairly normal, and a few are so sick they skip work during the final days.

Of course, with injections of human recombinant TSH, patients feel normal and complain only of the diet.

Once patients are prepared, the next step is to determine whether any thyroid remnants remain in the neck. To do this, we administer a trace dose of iodine, 80 to 100 microcuries of I-131 or 2–5 milicuries of I-123. Twenty-four hours later, we scan the neck with a gamma camera; 95 percent of the time, we observe some iodine absorption in the neck, which means there are thyroid remnants.

Next, we administer a therapeutic dose of radioactive iodine by capsule. Only iodine-131 can be used for treatment. Doses vary from center to center, between 30 and 150 millicuries. Typically at the Cleveland Clinic, we use 100 to 150 millicuries. This dosage will destroy all the thyroid remnants and the remaining cancer cells in most patients.

Since 5 percent of patients have no uptake in the neck when we give them the trace dose of iodine, they must have a whole body scan to check if there are any distant places where disease may have spread. If a patient is prepared by taking thyroid hormones and iodine-131 is used for the scan, the second, higher trace dosage is given (we give 2 millicuries). Forty-eight to 72 hours later, we scan the patient's entire body. If we see uptake in the neck or anywhere else, we administer a therapeutic dose to destroy the thyroid and/or cancer tissue.

If a patient is prepared by human recombinant TSH injections, we use only iodine-123 for the scan. Using this isotope allows us to perform a whole body scan 24 hours after the tracer dose is given and to make a final decision on the need for treatment while the TSH level is still high. Waiting 48–72 hours would result in TSH being in the 8–20 range.

If the body scan is negative, we stop treatment. Either that patient has had a perfect surgery (everything has been removed), or the cancer cannot absorb iodine.

Minimizing Recurrence

One therapeutic radioiodine dose should kill every thyroid remnant in the body within several weeks to several months after the treatment. The patient who was taken off the thyroid hormone resumes taking thyroid hormone supplements 24 to 48 hours after radioactive iodine therapy. Physicians prescribe a slightly higher thyroid hormone dose than is needed to treat the patient's hypothyroidism. This is done to suppress the TSH below the normal range (though not to the point where it is undetectable) to prevent any regrowth of the tumor if it is still present despite all the treatments. This approach has been proven to help minimize recurrence of the cancer.

Seven to ten days after radioactive iodine treatment, a whole body scan is performed. A gamma camera scans the patient from the top of the head to the tip of the toes. If the cancer has spread to any part of the body, the gamma camera will see it in the majority of cases. Usually, any remaining thyroid or cancer shows up in the neck. Occasionally, the scanner finds it in other parts of the body if it has metastasized. These cancer metastases will then be imaged by a CT or an MRI and treated with surgery if it is possible to excise or with external radiation if the location precludes operation.

Follow-Up Treatment for Well-Differentiated Thyroid Cancer

After radioactive iodine therapy, there must be adequate follow-up. Because patients who have had most or all of their thyroid removed will now be hypothyroid, they will have to take thyroid hormone for rest of their lives. But in these cases, treatment is not the same as for ordinary hypothyroid patients; we intentionally suppress the TSH, as mentioned before. So we start them on a dose that is slightly higher than what we calculate as the full replacement dose.

Patients differ in how much extra hormone is enough. Typically, the initial dosage needs to be tuned up or down. For this reason, the physician sees the patient about two months after treatment. At that time, we will measure the TSH and the free T4. The goal is to achieve a TSH between 0.4 and 0.05. If the TSH is higher than this, the dose of the thyroid hormone medication should be increased. If the TSH is completely suppressed, the dose should be lowered. The dosage should also be lowered a little if the patient has symptoms of hyperthyroidism. But this rarely happens.

During the same visit, the doctor will examine the patient's neck by palpation (touch). Physicians rarely discover any problems in the neck area during the first follow-up, but the neck should be examined at every opportunity. Some patients may complain of numbness in the scar area, but they usually have no other symptoms from the operation.

The next follow-up is four months later (six months after radioactive iodine treatment). At this time, we check TSH, which should still be in the desired range, and we test thyroglobulin and thyroglobulin antibody levels. The thyroglobulin antibody test will be positive in about 20 percent of the thyroid cancer population. As discussed in chapter 6, thyroglobulin antibodies distort thyroglobulin measurements. An accurate thyroglobulin measurement is extremely important because thyroglobulin is a protein that only thyroid cells produce. If patients are truly free of thyroid cells after surgery and radioactive iodine treatment, they will also be free of thyroglobulin. Any return of thyroglobulin would mean a return of thyroid cancer.

Unfortunately, the 20 percent who have thyroglobulin antibodies cannot fully benefit from this test and have to rely on other measurements to detect a recurrence of cancer. In the ideal situation, the patient has negative thyroglobulin antibodies and undetectable thyroglobulin.

If the patient has thyroglobulin antibodies or positive thyroglobulin, I perform an ultrasound exam of the neck, looking for any abnormal nodules that could signify the return of cancer. For patients who have negative thyroglobulin and thyroglobulin antibodies, I simply look at and touch the neck area at this appointment.

The next checkup should occur 9 to 12 months after the initial radioactive iodine treatment. This time, we optimize conditions for checking for any remaining or returning cancer. There are again two ways to prepare a patient for testing. One way is to take patients off thyroid hormone medication five weeks before their appointment. This will induce hypothyroidism and raise the TSH above 25. The elevated TSH will stimulate any remaining thyroid cancer cells to reveal themselves. The alternative is to give the patient two injections of synthetic TSH a day apart, which will elevate the TSH without inducing hypothyroidism.

There are also two ways of checking for cancer after the TSH has been upped. One is to measure the thyroglobulin blood level, but this method can be used only in people whose thyroglobulin antibodies are negative. If people have thyroglobulin antibodies, instead we scan the entire body with a radioactive iodine scan, using 2 to 5 millicuries of radioactive iodine.

If the cancer hasn't returned, the patient will have a negative scan and negative thyroglobulin. This occurs in about 90 percent of cases.

What if the Radioactive Iodine Scan Is Positive?

If the radioactive iodine scan is positive, we assume the cancer was never completely eliminated or that it has returned. With most patients, the remaining cancer will be in the neck. An ultrasound exam will determine whether the cancer is macroscopic (visible) or microscopic (so small that is impossible to detect by ultrasound).

Visible cancer should be removed by surgery whenever possible. If the ultrasound fails to show the cancer at the sites indicated by the scan, the physician will administer a larger dose of radioactive iodine, 100 to 300 millicuries, in a second attempt to kill the cancer remnants. Afterward, the patients will have the same follow-ups as after their initial treatments.

What Happens when the Thyroglobulin Test Is Positive?

A positive thyroglobulin test tells us only that cancer is present; it doesn't pinpoint the location of the disease. Since most recurrences occur in the neck, we first examine the neck with ultrasound. If we find abnormal tissue, we follow up with an FNA. If the FNA shows the tissue is malignant, a new surgery is ordered.

If the ultrasound shows nothing, patients are taken off thyroid medication (although some centers rely on synthetic TSH at this point) to boost their TSH level, then treated with radioactive iodine, 100 to 300 millicuries. This treatment will be followed seven to ten days later with a full-body scan, which will usually show the cancer sites. Again, in most cases, the cancer will be in the neck area (just too small to detect with ultrasound). But sometimes we find it in the lungs or bones and even more rarely in the liver, brain, and other locations.

Occasionally, patients with elevated thyroglobulin have negative whole body scans, even after high dose treatment. This means the cancer is not absorbing iodine. Some cancers actually lose their ability—or never have the ability—to pick up radioactive iodine. When we suspect cancer, but neck ultrasound and radioiodine scans are negative, we resort to a PET scan, which will usually show where the cancer is.

When found by a PET scan, the cancer can be treated and, hopefully, eradicated with surgery, radiation treatment, or if it is widespread, chemotherapy. But chemo is still only an experimental treatment for thyroid cancers.

If the PET scan is negative, we have run out of tools. At this point, we simply follow the patient's thyroglobulin levels. Often, these levels tend to stay the same. If they increase, we repeat the same evaluation procedures. Fortunately, these cases are rare, and most people in this category remain stable. If you can't find the cancer, it is because it is very small. Frequently, these cancers remain small for a long period. I have had only a couple of patients in this category.

If PET scans are so effective, why not use them right away and skip the other tests? There are several reasons a PET scan is used as a last resort:

1. PET scans are very expensive, about $5,000 per scan. (CT and MRI scans range from $200 to $800.)

2. Occasionally, PET scans produce false positive results, indicating cancer where there is none.

3. Thyroid cancers that absorb radioactive iodine are less likely to absorb the contrast agents used in PET scans. Similarly, thyroid cancers that PET scans can detect are frequently unable to absorb iodine.

What if the Radioactive Iodine Scan and Thyroglobulin Are Negative?

If both tests are negative, I will perform a neck ultrasound to rule out a rare case in which cancer does not take up iodine and does not make thyroglobulin. So far, I personally have not found any such cancers, but others have.

Those patients who, at the time of testing, have all tests negative and are cancer-free should be followed every six months with TSH and thyroglobulin tests for 3 to 5 years. At yearly intervals after radioactive iodine therapy, they should be given artificial TSH, then their thyroglobulin should be tested. This procedure should be repeated until 3 to 5 years after the surgery, and then every 2 years until 10 or 12 years have passed, and finally every 5 years for the remainder of the patient's life. If the cancer returns, the initial treatment should be repeated.

Thyroid cancers return in about 20 percent of patients. Usually, these recurrences happen in the first 5 years. But some recur more than 30 years after the original cancer was diagnosed. Both the patient and the physician must remain vigilant.

Are There Any Special Considerations?

If the cancer is very small, it may not be necessary to suppress the TSH (to prevent recurrence). It may be sufficient to maintain the TSH at the low end of the normal range (0.5–2.0).

For cancers that are more aggressive than usual (those that recur or have spread), the TSH should be suppressed to less than 0.05. Also, if the cancer is an aggressive type, a thyroglobulin test should be administered three months after the radioactive iodine treatment to make sure it is not progressing despite treatment.

Many experts recommend annual chest X-rays for thyroid cancer patients. I do not routinely prescribe chest X-rays because they frequently yield erroneous results, especially in older patients. I do, however, recommend chest X-rays when I suspect a recurrence of the cancer.

External radiation therapy entails delivering a beam of radiation energy from an X-ray machine or some other external source. This therapy is used when the physician cannot completely eliminate the cancer. It has been shown to delay progression of the disease.

Chemotherapy has thus far been disappointing in thyroid cancer treatment, though the chemo drug doxorubicin benefits about one-third of patients. New approaches are regularly being investigated.

Poorly Differentiated Thyroid Cancers

Not all thyroid cancers are easy to treat. In fact, the anaplastic thyroid cancer is one of the worst malignancies known. Luckily, these very aggressive cancers are rare.

Anaplastic Cancer

Unlike well-differentiated cancers (papillary and follicular), which are relatively easy to manage and have a consistent appearance under the microscope, poorly differentiated thyroid cancers like anaplastic cancer are unmanageable and have a jumbled appearance. This cancer is always considered advanced stage at diagnosis. While pathologists readily recognize the type and origin of well-differentiated cancers, they have a difficult time identifying poorly differentiated cancers and cannot determine their point of origin.

Like well-differentiated thyroid cancers, anaplastic thyroid cancers begin in the thyroid's follicular cells. But anaplastic cancer is extremely aggressive and spreads rapidly. Eighty percent of patients with anaplastic thyroid cancer die within a year of being diagnosed with the disease, even after aggressive treatment. Former Chief Justice William H. Rehnquist probably died from this type of thyroid cancer. He was diagnosed with thyroid cancer in October 2004 and died September 3, 2005, less than 11 months later. He was 80 years old.

Fortunately, anaplastic cancer is rare, representing 1 to 2 percent of all thyroid cancers. In the United States, about one to two individuals per million people develop this disease every year. Most of them are over 65; only 10 percent are younger than 50, and women are two to three times more likely to get it than men.

We do not know what causes this type of cancer, but roughly one in five anaplastic patients have already had a well-differentiated thyroid cancer. We suspect that most anaplastic cancers develop from well-differentiated cancers. Also, roughly half of these patients have a history of multinodular goiter. However, bear in mind that many patients have well-differentiated thyroid cancers, and even more have multinodular goiters, but only a small number ever develop anaplastic cancer.

How Do Doctors Detect Anaplastic Cancers? A lump on the neck that doubles or triples in size in a couple of weeks may signal the onset of anaplastic cancer. About 85 percent of anaplastic cancers are detected when patients notice a fast-growing mass in their necks. The mass usually consists of hard and soft bumps and is often fixed to surrounding tissue. Therefore, when a patient swallows, the lump doesn't budge.

The mass may also press against neighboring organs like the windpipe and esophagus, causing difficulty in breathing or swallowing. A third of patients have trouble breathing and/or swallowing, and 25 percent have hoarseness and/or a cough. Sometimes patients with anaplastic cancer are given a tracheostomy (a hole is surgically cut in the windpipe) to facilitate breathing.

A biopsy (FNA or other forms) confirms the diagnosis.

A CT scan of the neck and chest is used to measure the cancer's size and detect invasion of the cancer into neck and chest structures, like the esophagus and lungs. We also use a bone scan and X-rays to detect skeletal spread. Unfortunately, in about 90 percent of patients, the cancer has already invaded surrounding tissue or spread to other parts of the body at the time of diagnosis. The metastasis occurs most often in the lungs (90 percent of patients), bones (up to 15 percent of patients), and brain (about 5 percent of patients).

How Is Anaplastic Cancer Treated? Surgery is the best option if the tumor is small (less than 5 centimeters). Unfortunately, most patients are not candidates for curative surgery because the disease has already spread beyond the neck when it is discovered. But if the tumor hasn't spread, it can be removed without excising the entire thyroid. The survival rate is not affected by leaving some thyroid tissue intact. Sometimes, patients undergo surgery just to get relief from difficulties breathing and swallowing.

In addition, radiation therapy and chemotherapy may be used to shrink the tumor and prolong survival; but in general, these are not very effective treatments with this type of cancer. Twenty-five percent of patients will survive for two years if the tumor is less than 6 centimeters. The two-year survival rate for larger tumors is 15 percent.

Advanced anaplastic tumor with metastasis is virtually always deadly, and no effective therapy exists.

Medullary Thyroid Cancer

Medullary thyroid cancer is different from previously described tumors in many ways. Most important, it develops in the C cells (parafollicular cells) of the thyroid, which live between the thyroid follicles.

While the follicular cells of the thyroid develop from the tissue at the base of the tongue, the C cells evolve from neural tissue, as do the brain and nerves. As the thyroid gland develops in the fetus, the C cells migrate into the thyroid. In spite of their location, C cells have no thyroid function. They are more or less squatter cells just looking for a place to live. C cells do some work; they produce calcitonin, a hormone that contributes to calcium regulation in some animals. But in humans, this hormone has very little effect on calcium levels. Removal of all the C cells in humans has no adverse effect on calcium levels or metabolism. In fact, it has no known clinical significance. In human beings, the only role C cells seem to have is as a source for medullary cancers.

About 80 percent of medullary cancers are sporadic; that is, they occur randomly in people. The rest are called familial and develop among members of the same family. Medullary cancers are distributed equally between men and women.

The familial form is unique among cancers. Virtually all patients with familial medullary cancer have a mutation of a gene called RET proto-oncogene. This mutated gene is found in all the cells of their bodies. In fact, several dozen different mutations have been discovered in this gene; each of the mutations predispose the people who carry them to develop medullary thyroid cancers. These people are prone to develop benign tumors in the adrenal and parathyroid glands as well. Only malignant tumors occurring in these individuals is medullary cancer.

Half of the patients with sporadic medullary cancer have this same gene mutation, but it is found only in their medullary cancer cells, not in the other cells of their bodies. The most important difference between sporadic and familial medullary cancer is that people with the familial form can pass the mutation on to their children since all their cells are affected, even sperm and ova. People with the sporadic form cannot pass it on to their children.

When patients are diagnosed with medullary thyroid cancer, they must be tested for all the known gene mutations. We do this by analyzing the white blood cells. If a mutation is discovered, a patient's family members must be tested for the same mutations. If any of them test positive, their thyroids will be removed, which will prevent them from ever developing any form of this cancer. But occasionally, some family members will already have medullary cancer in their thyroids. They should be treated as any other patient with medullary thyroid carcinoma (see page 161). If no mutations are detected in the initial case, the patient does not have the familial form of the disease, and other family members do not need to be tested.

How Is Medullary Thyroid Cancer Detected? Medullary thyroid cancer is usually detected as a solitary thyroid nodule in the upper part of the thyroid lobes, where the C cells are most abundant. Following detection, the doctor biopsies the patient with an

FNA, and the pathologist will make a diagnosis. Most patients with sporadic cancer are over 50, while most people with the familial form are under 30.

After an FNA diagnosis, we stage the medullary thyroid cancer by administering an ultrasound or CT examination of the neck and an X-ray of the chest, followed by a CT if any abnormality is detected. CT scans are excellent at detecting the spread of the cancer in most cases.

In 50 percent of all patients, the cancer has spread to the neck lymph nodes at the time of detection. Approximately 12.5 percent experience some difficulty breathing or swallowing, or their voices change because of cancer spreading into the surrounding tissue. In 5 percent of cases, the cancer will have metastasized beyond the neck.

Like C cells, medullary tumors produce calcitonin; therefore, patients with medullary cancer have high calcitonin blood levels. Before the RET proto-oncogene mutations were discovered, doctors relied on calcitonin measurements to detect familial medullary cancer in family members.

Medullary tumors also frequently manufacture a substance called carcinoembryonic antigen (CEA), as well as other substances that can cause bouts of diarrhea and flushing (similar to menopausal hot flashes). A high level of CEA and calcitonin in the blood are the markers for the disease presence. Medullary cancer can also stimulate the adrenal glands to produce too many steroids. This occurs only in advanced stages of cancer.

Staging Medullary Cancer. In cases of medullary cancer, staging can be done prior to surgery (rather than afterward, as with well-differentiated cancer).

Stages are assigned as follows:

Stage 1: The thyroid tumor is smaller than 2 centimeters, and there are no signs of metastasis or local invasion.

Stage 2: The tumor is between 2 and 4 centimeters, and there are no signs of metastasis or local invasion (the tumor is confined to the thyroid gland).

Stage 3: The tumor is larger than 4 centimeters, or there are smaller tumors in which the cancer has spread to the local lymph nodes (those closest to the thyroid gland).

Stage 4: There is a tumor of any size accompanied by metastasis to lymph nodes other than those closest to the thyroid, there is any metastasis to distant sites, or there is local invasion of the tumor into surrounding tissue.

The higher the stage, the worse the prognosis. Patients with stages 3 and 4 usually survive three to five years. Patients under 40 years of age have better survival rates than older people.

Other Evaluations. Before patients who have the RET proto-oncogene mutation undergo surgery for medullary thyroid cancer, they must be evaluated for other conditions that accompany the familial form of the disease, as mentioned above. Most important, the physician needs to measure calcium levels in the blood. About one-third of patients have a tumor in one of their parathyroid glands, which causes elevated levels of calcium. Parathyroid tumors can be cut out during the cancer surgery.

Physicians need to also test to see whether the patient has a rare form of adrenal tumor called pheochromocytoma. A pheochromocytoma, or "pheo" tumor, is common in patients with medullary cancer.

A pheo tumor secretes epinephrine (adrenaline) and norepinephrine, causing attacks of high blood pressure, sweating, anxiety, heart palpitations, and severe headaches. If it is not treated, it can cause severe problems during surgery. Anesthesia may cause the tumor to release large amounts of epinephrine and norepinephrine, causing dangerously unstable blood pressure and even death. Pheo tumors must be removed prior to cancer surgery. Patients will be prescribed medications for a few weeks to prepare them for pheo surgery.

Before surgery, doctors will measure calcitonin and carcinoembryonic antigen levels. After surgery, they will measure these levels again and compare the values to the earlier ones.

Surgical Treatment for Poorly Differentiated Thyroid Cancer

Total thyroidectomy is the preferred surgical treatment for poorly differentiated thyroid cancer for several reasons:

- Roughly 30 percent of sporadic cases and all familial patients harbor multiple tumors in their thyroids. The only way to be sure all the tumors are cut out is by removing the entire thyroid gland.

- Also, patients who have a mutation in the RET proto-oncogene must have all their C cells removed; otherwise, they will eventually develop another medullary thyroid cancer.

During surgery, the surgeon will examine and remove all lymph nodes next to the thyroid gland. Nodes that are farther away will be examined, and suspicious ones will be removed.

After the thyroid is removed, the patient must immediately begin thyroid hormone replacement therapy. But for this type of thyroid cancer, there is no need to suppress the TSH (as with papillary and follicular thyroid cancers) because the TSH level does not affect C cells. Therefore, the physician will prescribe a dose that normalizes the thyroid function. Calcium levels must be checked because they can drop abnormally low. Some patients will have permanent hypoparathyroidism (lack of parathyroid hormone, which is the principal regulator of blood calcium levels). The patients in whom calcium levels drop below normal must be given vitamin D and calcium supplements to keep them safe.

Patients with medullary thyroid cancer are never treated with radioactive iodine because C cells do not pick up iodine.

The calcitonin and CEA levels in the blood should be measured six months after surgery. If all the C cells have been successfully removed, calcitonin should be undetectable. However, calcitonin frequently remains positive even when all the C cells are gone. This is because the high level of calcitonin prior to surgery led to its deposition all around the body in different tissues. After the surgery, this calcitonin leaks back to circulation, and some level of calcitonin is maintained in the blood for years, even though disease is eradicated. In addition, often some C cells remain after the surgery; thus, in both scenarios the calcitonin level is much lower but still detectable in most patients. CEA should be within normal levels. When both CEA and calcitonin are within normal range six months after surgery, medullary cancer usually doesn't return. (Otherwise, about 5 percent will recur over the next five years.)

Afterward, calcitonin and CEA are measured every six months. If, six months after surgery, the calcitonin rises or remains over 100 picograms per milliliter, the physician should search for residual cancer with an ultrasound of the neck and a CT scan of the chest and abdomen. If nothing is found, the doctor will follow up with a whole body scan using Indium-111 pentetreotide, a special scan that may find abnormal tissue in 60 to 70 percent of cases.

The bones should also be scanned using bone-specific radioactive contrast because sometimes metastasis from medullary thyroid cancer will be in the skeleton.

If the cancer still isn't detected, the doctor will refer the patient to a tertiary center, where more aggressive searches can be done. These methods include sampling blood from the veins of individual organs. The blood is then analyzed for calcitonin and CEA. If there is a vein that has high concentrations of these, the doctor knows that the tumor is somewhere in the area that is drained by this particular vein. A microdissection of that area can then be performed.

If these measures fail to reveal cancer, the surgeon will perform microdissection of the neck and upper chest hoping to remove all tumor tissue.

If a patient's calcitonin is over 1,000 picograms per milliliter, the patient will most likely have distant spread (metastasis) of the disease, usually in the liver.

Patients with widespread medullary cancer can be temporarily helped by chemotherapy using the drugs doxorubicin and dacarbazine. When there is no hope for a cure, the patient is given external radiation treatments, which delay progression of the disease but can't arrest it.

Lymphomas

Thyroid lymphoma is yet another tumor that originates in the thyroid. But it doesn't arise from thyroid cells. All lymphomas develop from lymphocytes, the immune cells that patrol the body. These rare tumors make up about 2 percent of all thyroid tumors.

We know of only one factor that increases a person's chance of developing thyroid lymphoma: preexisting Hashimoto's thyroiditis. Lymphoma is 60 to 75 times more common in people with thyroiditis. Most people who get it are over the age of 60, and women, who are more prone to Hashimoto's, develop the disease much more often than men do.

Thyroid lymphoma is usually accompanied by a rapidly growing thyroid goiter. Patients frequently have problems with breathing, swallowing, and hoarseness. About one in ten has what are called B symptoms—fever, night sweats, and weight loss—which are characteristic of all types of lymphoma.

The disease is usually diagnosed with an FNA, but sometimes we can't tell whether the patient has ordinary Hashimoto's thyroiditis or lymphoma. In such cases, a special analysis is required, which may include a coarse needle aspiration or an open surgical biopsy.

How Do Doctors Stage Thyroid Lymphoma?

To stage thyroid lymphoma, physicians usually use the staging system developed at the University of Michigan at Ann Arbor:

Stage 1: The disease is limited to the thyroid, which occurs in about 50 percent of cases.

Stage 2: The disease is limited to the thyroid and local lymph nodes, which occurs in about 45 percent of patients.

Stage 3: The cancer has spread to the lymph nodes on both sides of the diaphragm (the primary breathing muscle located between chest and abdomen), in 2 to 3 percent of patients.

Stage 4: The cancer has spread to other organs on both sides of the diaphragm, in 2 to 3 percent of patients.

How Is Thyroid Lymphoma Treated?

Surgery can cure the patient only when the disease is contained in the thyroid gland. In advanced cases, breathing can be so difficult that a tracheostomy must be performed.

Fortunately, these tumors are very sensitive to radiation and chemotherapy. External radiation is the primary therapy for stages 1 and 2 and will control the cancer in about 75 percent of patients. A little chemotherapy further improves results. Such combination therapy is becoming the standard of care.

Patients with advanced lymphomas (stages 3 and 4) are usually treated with chemotherapy alone, as are patients whose cancer returns after radiation treatment. There are many protocols for chemotherapy; but at this time, it is not clear which is the best.

Approximately 85 percent of patients with stages 1 and 2 achieve complete remission after their initial treatment. About one-half of them relapse in five years. The five-year survival is 80 percent for stage 1 and about 55 percent for stage 2. For stages 3 and 4, it is between 15 and 35 percent.

We frequently tell our patients that thyroid cancer is the "best cancer you can get," and it is true in about 95 percent of cases. Unfortunately, sometimes it is not true and the disease is progressive despite our treatments. But even in these patients, the course of the disease is often protracted and they live many years before the disease catches up with them.

Chapter 9

Pregnancy and Your Thyroid

P regnancy does not cause thyroid disease; but in the beginning, it can lead to some changes in the thyroid's functioning:

- It causes the production of more thyroid hormones.

- It stimulates production of thyroid-binding globulin.

- It may enlarge the thyroid temporarily because of relative iodine deficiency.

Let's take a closer look at how conception affects the thyroid.

Pregnancy produces changes in the metabolism to which the thyroid gland must adapt. In the early stages of pregnancy, the body manufactures large amounts of a hormone called human chorionic gonadotropin (HCG). This hormone, which is similar to TSH, attaches to the TSH receptors on thyroid cells and stimulates production of thyroid hormones.

But hormone production rarely exceeds normal levels because the pituitary compensates by decreasing the amount of TSH it makes. This can be so pronounced that TSH will fall below the normal level, leading doctors to mistake the woman's condition

Planning a Pregnancy

If you have well-controlled hypothyroidism, be sure to inform your doctor if you become pregnant. Most women will need a dosage adjustment in their T4 prescription because of an increase in TBG levels, the same kind of adjustment normal thyroids would make.

for hyperthyroidism and erroneously prescribe antithyroid medication.

Pregnancy also stimulates production of thyroid-binding globulin, or TBG, the protein that binds thyroid hormones in the bloodstream. Having higher levels of TBG means more of the thyroid hormone in the bloodstream will be bound, leaving less as free hormone. In addition, these binding proteins break down more slowly than normal during pregnancy.

The combined effect of these two changes can increase the amount of TBG in the blood to twice its normal level. The pituitary gland (the supervisor) senses these changes and orders the thyroid to work harder by sending more TSH. The thyroid gland responds by increasing thyroid hormone production to maintain the free levels of T4 and T3 within normal range. The new balance is reached, and the mother-to-be remains healthy.

Many women become moderately iodine deficient during pregnancy due to an increased elimination of iodine in the urine. This causes the thyroid to grow. In the United States, the average size increase of a thyroid during pregnancy is 18 percent. This enlargement is normal and does not require treatment. After delivery, the gland returns to its normal size.

Pregnancy and Preexisting Conditions

Because pregnancy can affect the thyroid, it may also trigger or emphasize any preexisting thyroid conditions. If you are a woman planning a pregnancy or you are already pregnant and you suspect you may have a thyroid disorder, if you know thyroid disorders run in your family, or if you have been experiencing any of the symptoms for hypothyroidism and hyperthyroidism listed in chapters 2 and 4, it is extremely important that you talk to your doctor.

Heather

Heather was extremely anxious. She had just learned she was pregnant—for the fourth time in three years. But she didn't have any children. Her first three pregnancies had ended in miscarriages within the first two to three months. Her doctors couldn't figure out why.

On her own, Heather had learned that thyroid abnormalities may cause spontaneous abortion. So she asked her doctor for a referral to see a specialist to reevaluate her thyroid, which he had diagnosed as healthy.

When Heather came to her appointment with me, she constantly shifted in her seat and fidgeted. I asked whether any members of her family had thyroid conditions. "My mother is hypothyroid," she said, brightening. "Could that be why I haven't had a baby?"

It was too early to tell, so I asked whether other family members had thyroid diseases. "No," Heather replied. "My sisters, nephews, and nieces are all healthy." Suddenly, she reached for my hand and said, "Doctor, please, I want this baby! Help me. Something must be wrong with my thyroid. Something must be messed up."

She had her medical records with her, but as I reviewed them, I saw no abnormalities. Her TSH had been in the normal range for each pregnancy—4.1, 3.9, and 4.2 milliunits per milliliter, respectively. Her free T4 and T3 were also normal, though a bit on the low side.

I didn't think her thyroid had caused the miscarriages. Nevertheless, I checked her antimicrosomal antibody level and assured her I would do whatever I could to determine whether or not a thyroid problem had caused the miscarriages.

Two days later, when Heather's results came back, I was surprised to learn that her antimicrosomal antibody level was high. This showed me she had Hashimoto's thyroiditis. When expecting women have any thyroid disorder, we call it maternal thyroid disease, but the condition is not caused by pregnancy—it just happens to occur in a woman who is pregnant.

Maternal thyroid diseases can cause miscarriage, future infertility, early delivery, low birth weight, stillbirth, heart failure in the mother, and intellectual deficiencies in babies. Also, the infants of women with under- or overactive thyroids may be born hypothyroid or hyperthyroid. It is easy to see the importance of treating any thyroid disease in a pregnant woman.

I prescribed T4 supplementation to decrease Heather's TSH to the low side of the normal range, between 1.0 and 2.0 milliunits per milliliter. I advised her to call me at once if any signs of hyperthyroidism developed or if she experienced pregnancy-related problems. We scheduled to meet in a month. (Normally, I would wait two months, but to calm Heather's anxiety, I decided to check in sooner.)

Heather's research was right: hypothyroidism often causes miscarriages within the first three months of pregnancy. That is why it is rare to see advanced pregnancies complicated by hypothyroidism. Miscarriages are also attributed to high levels of antithyroid antibodies, like those Heather had, even when thyroid hormone levels and TSH are still within normal range.

When Heather returned in a month, she felt healthy and hopeful. She was still pregnant. Her TSH had dropped to 2.74 milliunits per milliliter, and her free T4 and T3 had climbed to the upper half of the normal range. So I kept her on the same dose of T4 and made an appointment to see her again in a month.

A month later, her TSH level had fallen further, to under 2.0. For the next six months, we maintained her TSH below 2.0. At the end of that period, she gave birth to a healthy baby boy, Ryan.

This is just one case, so speaking absolutely scientifically, we can't be certain that the treatment was responsible for her successful pregnancy. But I think it helped, and Heather is convinced it did.

I suspect that when Heather first came in, she was in the early stages of hypothyroidism, and it had nothing to do with her being pregnant. Her TSH level, which was on the high end of the normal range, was not ideal for her. Therefore, she now continues to take T4 after pregnancy (although at a somewhat lower dose). She is currently feeling healthy, so I will continue to maintain her TSH level at just under 2.0 milliunits per milliliter.

What if I'm Hypothyroid?

If you have well-controlled hypothyroidism, you must inform your doctor if you become pregnant. Most women in this situation will need a dosage adjustment in their T4 prescription because normal thyroids would adjust T4 levels. The usual increase in dose is about 30 percent.

After delivery, the physician should lower the T4 dose for hypothyroid women to pre-pregnancy levels. The TSH should be tested six to eight weeks after giving birth. Any fine-tuning of their dosage should be done at this time.

Adequately treated hypothyroid mothers excrete only small amounts of thyroid hormones in their milk (the same as mothers without any thyroid dysfunction); therefore, breast-feeding is safe for both the mother and the baby.

If you get pregnant, have your thyroid checked between the fourth and sixth week of pregnancy. If the results are normal, you don't need to have your thyroid checked again. But if any abnormality is found, your thyroid should be rechecked every three months throughout the pregnancy.

Even mild uncontrolled hypothyroidism during pregnancy may affect the neuropsychological development of a baby. Studies show slightly lower IQ scores in seven- to nine-year-olds whose mothers had elevated TSH levels during pregnancy than in children whose mothers did not have elevated TSH.

Most of the children's IQs were still within the normal range, though some fell below normal. Fifteen percent of the children whose mothers had elevated TSH had below-normal IQs, while only 5 percent of children whose mothers had normal TSH had IQs that were below normal.

Risks of Hypothyroidism in Mothers-to-Be

It is essential to ensure a normal thyroid hormone supply during pregnancy for several reasons:

- To avoid symptoms of hypothyroidism in the mother
- To prevent miscarriage
- Because the baby's development could be affected by the mother's hypothyroidism

Even if a hypothyroid mother doesn't miscarry, an underactive thyroid causes other complications during pregnancy. These problems occur even more often with severe hypothyroidism.

Complications of Pregnancy and Hypothyroidism. If hypothyroidism is untreated or undertreated during pregnancy, a number of complications can occur, including:

- Elevation of the mother's blood pressure
- Placental abruption (separation of the placenta from the uterus)
- Early delivery
- Low birth weight
- Increased risk of infant death during or shortly after delivery
- Increased bleeding after delivery
- Increased risk of affecting the baby's neuropsychological development

Who Should Be Tested?

Professional organizations of gynecologists, obstetricians, and endocrinologists do not currently recommend routine thyroid testing of women who intend to become pregnant. But I do test all women with even slight symptoms that could be attributed to thyroid disease, as well as those who have a family history of thyroid disease or a personal history of any other autoimmune disorder.

All pregnant women should have their thyroids checked between the fourth and sixth week of pregnancy. If the results are normal, they don't need to have their thyroid checked again. But if any abnormality is found, their thyroid should be rechecked every three months throughout the pregnancy.

What if I Am Hyperthyroid?

When the placenta secretes human chorionic gonadotropin in the early stages of pregnancy, it can stimulate the TSH receptors in the thyroid. This causes 10 to 20 percent of healthy pregnant women to have short-term, low-level hyperthyroidism. This is a normal condition and does not require treatment.

Unfortunately, it can be hard to tell the difference between symptoms of true hyperthyroidism and those of a normal pregnancy. In either case, a woman may experience excessive sweating, feel constantly warm, be nervous, vomit, and have heart palpitations.

But there are two symptoms that occur in hyperthyroid women that healthy pregnant women do not normally have: weight loss and an accelerated heartbeat of more than 100 beats per minute. Pregnant women with either or both of these symptoms should seek medical help immediately because this may indicate the presence of hyperthyroidism, which should be treated. About 0.2 percent of pregnant women are found to be hyperthyroid.

Some women develop an abnormal abundance of placental tissue (hydatidiform mole) during early pregnancy or a malignant tumor called choriocarcinoma. These are rare conditions, but in both of them, excess human chorionic gonadotropin is produced and may cause hyperthyroidism. However, no specific therapy is needed for the hyperthyroidism. Instead, the hydatidiform mole must be surgically removed and the choriocarcinoma treated appropriately as a malignant tumor. Sadly, in both cases, the fetus will not survive.

Full-blown hyperthyroidism in pregnancy is triggered by the usual causes—Graves' disease, thyroid nodules, and inflammation of thyroiditis, as well as other rare causes—and is accompanied by a low TSH.

Tricky to Diagnose

Since TSH can also be slightly low in normal pregnancies, it is not always easy to recognize hyperthyroidism in early pregnancy. In addition, the total T4 and T3 may be elevated in normal pregnancies because of the natural increase in thyroid-binding globulin levels described above. An accurate diagnosis of full-fledged hyperthyroidism in pregnancy should therefore be based on a TSH reading below 0.01 milliunits per milliliter and an elevated free T4 and/or T3 (not total values).

Finding the Cause

Diagnosing the cause of the hyperthyroidism is complicated during pregnancy. We cannot use the standard radioactive iodine tests because the developing thyroid tissue in the fetus would also pick up the radioactive iodine. Developing tissues are much more sensitive to injury by radioactivity than already developed adult tissue.

The most common cause is Graves' disease, which is accompanied by elevated levels of TSH receptor antibodies (thyroid receptor antibodies). This makes a diagnosis of Graves' disease easy to confirm by a thyroid receptor antibodies test.

Treating with PTU

With some pregnant patients, it is impossible to determine the cause of the hyperthyroidism during the pregnancy. In these cases, we treat patients with propylthiouracil (PTU) three times per day. But the PTU dosage, which is based on the patient's free T4 level, must be kept low for the safety of the baby. PTU can navigate from the mother through the placenta into the baby's system. If the infant absorbs too much PTU, its thyroid, which becomes active in the tenth week of pregnancy, won't produce sufficient hormone. These children may be born hypothyroid, without enough hormones to support normal development. Some babies develop a goiter when their mothers are treated with PTU at too high a dosage.

For these reasons, we don't try to normalize the free T4 level completely. Instead, we maintain it on the high end of the normal range and even little higher than normal, using the lowest possible PTU dosage necessary to alleviate maternal symptoms.

One to five percent of the children of women with Graves' disease during pregnancy are born hyperthyroid because the mother's thyroid-stimulating antibodies travel into the fetal bloodstream and overstimulate the baby's thyroid. Infants with this disorder may have increased heart rate, goiter, poor physical growth, and abnormal bone development. All babies of hyperthyroid mothers should be checked for hyperthyroidism immediately after delivery.

Fortunately, the baby's body gradually destroys the mother's antibodies within a few months after delivery, so the hyperthyroidism is only transient. However, hyperthyroid infants must be treated with antithyroid medications during this period to ensure normal growth and development.

After learning about the risks their newborns face, some hyperthyroid mothers resist treatment for their condition. But if maternal hyperthyroidism goes untreated, the trauma of labor could unleash a thyroid storm—a potentially fatal situation if not treated immediately.

Mothers who continue taking PTU after delivery should not breast-feed their babies; PTU is excreted into the milk and can cause hypothyroidism in the child. Also, if you are treated after delivery with radioactive iodine for hyperthyroidism, breast-feeding is absolutely out of the question.

A handful of women are allergic to PTU, and the only treatment option then becomes surgical removal of the thyroid. The timing of this surgery depends on the severity of the woman's condition. Generally, it is safest to operate between the fourth and seventh months of pregnancy.

Thyroid Treatment Before Getting Pregnant

Women who have been treated with radioactive iodine or thyroid surgery prior to pregnancy may continue to produce thyroid-stimulating antibodies long after their treatment, and their babies may be affected even though the mothers are no longer hyperthyroid. Babies born to mothers in this situation should be carefully monitored for increased heart rate; and if necessary, antithyroid medications can be prescribed.

How Does Thyroid Cancer Affect Pregnancy?

When a thyroid nodule is discovered during pregnancy, it should be evaluated in the same manner as any other nodule (see chapter 7), except that a radioactive iodine scan cannot be administered. If the nodule is cancerous, it should be removed by surgery.

The fact that most thyroid cancers grow slowly often allows physicians to postpone surgery until after birth. A study that tracked mothers with thyroid cancer for 20 years after they gave birth found that their survival rate was unaffected by the timing of their surgery.

Fortunately, thyroid cancer does not affect fetal development, and the babies are born healthy.

Are There Other Considerations I Should Be Aware Of?

Postpartum Depression

Postpartum depression affects 10 to 15 percent of women, and thyroid dysfunction occurs in about 10 percent of women after giving birth. When the disorders occur together, the symptoms of depression can be aggravated by the hypothyroidism.

However, people often assume that new mothers who are actually suffering from underactive thyroids are solely going through postpartum depression. All women who suffer from depression after giving birth should be tested for thyroid dysfunction. If hypothyroidism is detected, it should be treated in the standard manner. The thyroid hormone replacement therapy will help alleviate the woman's depression and improve her overall health and stamina.

Postpartum Thyroiditis

About 8 to 10 percent of women have postpartum thyroiditis. Most cases are mild and display no symptoms. Most have the same antithyroid antibodies in the bloodstream that we find in Hashimoto's thyroiditis (antimicrosomal and antithyroglobulin antibodies). Also, they are more likely to develop permanent hypothyroidism than are individuals with silent thyroiditis.

This form of thyroiditis is likely to occur again with the next pregnancy and may aggravate problems with postpartum depression.

Since Graves' disease can also start after delivery, it is important to distinguish between these conditions because the treatment is radically different.

Important Advice for All Mothers

Every woman who has a baby should have a thyroid test about six weeks after giving birth to assess the health of her thyroid gland and undergo any necessary treatment.

Chapter 10

Thyroid Controversies

Where Experts Disagree

Thyroid treatment is not always black and white. There are gray areas in which even the experts do not agree on what constitutes appropriate or inappropriate therapy. Also, some treatments are helpful for some patients but harmful to others. Often, the best therapy can only be determined on a case-by-case basis. In addition, people today have access to vast amounts of medical information in the popular press and on the Internet. Much of this information is unproven, some is misleading, and some can be dangerous. This has led to a great deal of uncertainty as to which treatments are best and which might be harmful. I always try to help my patients know and understand what I believe are the best, safest, and most effective options for them.

I decided to include this chapter as a place to present the latest findings on these controversial topics and treatments, as well as to express my opinions and current practices pertaining to them.

Controversy #1: Using Thyroid Hormones for Weight Loss

Taking thyroid hormone to lose weight is a very dangerous weight-loss program.

America has gotten fat during the last 50 years or so. Dieting and exercising are national obsessions. Yet less than 5 percent of overweight people shed significant weight and keep it off for more than a year.

Many believe their weight gain doesn't tally with their eating habits. Those who count calories and relentlessly work out often feel that weight loss doesn't reflect their rigorous dieting regimen and exercise routine.

The thyroid has become a convenient scapegoat. *My metabolism is just slow* is a common argument. *If I were a little more hyper, I could thin out.*

While it is true that hypothyroidism may stimulate a slight weight gain, the expanding American waistline cannot be attributed to a national epidemic of hypothyroidism and sluggish metabolisms. Most weight gain has nothing to do with the thyroid gland. Our metabolisms haven't uniformly slowed down. The simple truth is that Americans have become more sedentary.

Is Weight Gain My Thyroid's Fault?

Despite medical fact, many websites tout the idea that weight gain is rooted in thyroid dysfunction that traditional medical tests fail to diagnose. Many people desperately try to rev up their metabolisms in a last-ditch effort to lose weight by ingesting thyroid hormones. They are rarely successful, and most of them don't have thyroid disease. At least, not yet.

Hypothyroidism does put the brakes on the metabolism. But slowing the metabolism mainly affects the body at rest, not in action, and it should not cause major weight gain. Hypothyroid people require as much fuel to perform a task as do people with healthy thyroids. In other words, it takes the same amount of effort for a hypothyroid person to lift a 50-pound sack as it does a healthy person.

But hypothyroid people are more easily fatigued, which makes carrying out daily chores more difficult. If they do less and eat the same amount, they will gain weight. However, when hypothyroid people force themselves to maintain daily activities, as many do, weight gain rarely exceeds ten pounds. Of course, the longer treatment is delayed, the more pounds people put on.

But patients who believe their fat will melt away once they control their hypothyroidism are deluding themselves. Very few patients shed weight easily after normalizing their thyroid hormone levels. When people don't lose as much as they expect, many insist their doctors increase the T4 dosage. The doctor must severely overtreat them if they are going to lose weight simply by taking thyroid hormones. Such a therapy would lead to hyperthyroidism, and the patients would suffer from many of those symptoms and be at risk for heart failure. Also, patients would lose not merely fat but muscle mass as well.

What About Energy Levels?

Another reason patients believe they need to up their T4 dosage is that they often don't feel as energetic as they did before the onset of hypothyroidism. This is usually partly attributable to their weight gain. If you carry an additional 20 to 30 pounds all day, you won't feel as frisky, and you'll need to rest more often.

On the upside, patients who put on weight because of hypothyroidism usually have no problems keeping it off—once they lose it. But shedding it takes work: consistent exercise and dieting.

Relatively recent research suggests that the body's natural reaction to weight loss is to decrease T3 levels in the blood. We also know that the body converts a smaller quantity of T4 into T3 when people are under stress from trauma or severe illness. These parallel discoveries led doctors to prescribe T3 supplementation to both overweight and severely ill patients, believing that normalizing T3 levels would help the former lose weight and the latter recover more quickly. However, it turns out that adding T3 to weight-loss medications may cause adverse effects, and that giving severely ill patients T3 supplements actually worsens their condition.

Well, How Do I Manage My Weight Without Thyroid Medication?

The principles of weight management are simple. If you take in more energy than you burn, you gain weight. If you burn more than you absorb, you lose weight. Simple as it is to understand this principle, it is very hard to apply on a permanent basis in real life. It is easy to do it in the short run, but to really be successful, one needs to make permanent changes in energy intake and energy expenditure.

Food energy is measured in calories, a widely used term that is just as widely misunderstood. One calorie is the amount of energy required to raise the temperature of 1 gram of water from 15 degrees Celsius to 16 degrees Celsius. This is a minuscule unit of energy. When you eat 1 gram of sugar (about one-fourth of a teaspoon), you absorb 4,100 calories! Shocked? What we call a *calorie* in common parlance is actually 1,000 calories, or 1 kilocalorie. If a food or beverage label claims that one serving (one cup) has 200 calories, it actually contains 200 kilocalories or 200,000 calories!

How much energy do our daily diets provide? Sugars and proteins contain 4.1 kilocalories per gram (about 1,800 kilocalories per pound). Fat packs energy much more densely—9.1 kilocalories per gram (4,100 kilocalories per pound). Alcohol has about 7 kilocalories per gram (about 3,200 kilocalories per pound).

How many calories can someone consume in a day and still lose weight? The most reliable clinical studies come from metabolic chamber research. A subject is confined inside a metabolic chamber (a small, controlled room) for 24 hours in complete isolation. Under such conditions, we can precisely tally energy expenditure by controlling calorie intake and measuring the oxygen the subject uses as well as his or her carbon dioxide production.

Research shows that no adult, regardless of size or age, can maintain weight if he or she eats 1,200 kilocalories or less per day. (Of course, a large person will be able to ingest more calories than a small person and still lose weight.)

This seems a deceptively easy regimen to follow. But in fact, people notoriously underestimate the number of calories they ingest. In one study, subjects were told to eat 1,600 kilocalories per day. They averaged 2,200 kilocalories!

Similarly, people are prone to overestimate the number of calories they burn through exercise. If a 150-pound person walks one mile, he or she uses up between 80 and 100 kilocalories. You have to walk more than a mile to shed the calories in one serving of fat-free plain yogurt!

One pound of fat tissue contains 3,700 kilocalories of energy. (The figure is lower than that of pure fat because fat tissue is composed of not only fat but also blood, blood vessels, and so forth.) The same 150-pound person would have to walk 37 miles to burn off a pound of fat. Shedding ten pounds is a much longer hike— 370 miles!

Losing weight isn't as simple as it seems; nevertheless, it is the easiest part of weight management. The hardest part is keeping it off. This usually requires a 180-degree lifestyle shift.

Most weight-loss programs treat obesity as an acute illness. But obesity is not a typical illness like a lung infection. You can't cure it with a pill or a series of treatments. It is a lifelong condition that requires lifelong treatment.

Controversy #2: Prescribing Combination Therapy

Today, combination T4 and T3 therapy is controversial, but it was once standard treatment for hypothyroidism. It came into use in 1891 when sheep thyroid extract was first injected into a myxedema patient. Sheep thyroid, of course, contains both T4 and T3. Even after T4 was successfully synthesized in 1927 and became commercially available in 1949, physicians continued to use combination therapy. But since the 1970s, when it was discovered that the body converts T4 into T3, T4 has become the preferred treatment method. It allows for easier dosing than combination therapy, and it stabilizes the blood levels of both T4 and T3.

But interest in combination therapy has not disappeared. Because a few patients never feel as good as they did before becoming hypothyroid, some practitioners believe these people need T3 supplementation in addition to T4. Other doctors (and many practitioners of alternative medicine) simply believe that all patients should be treated with combination therapy.

Does Combination Therapy Really Help?

My clinical experience tells me that most patients can be successfully treated with only T4. But in a minority of people, some hypothyroid symptoms persist after treatment. In these cases, it is difficult to determine whether the patient's problems are related to thyroid function or other factors, such as poor sleeping patterns, weight gain, side effects from other medications, depression, stress, or diseases with similar symptoms.

I have tried combination therapy with several hundred patients. In most cases, it didn't help, but a few people clearly benefited. However, I have no way of knowing in advance who these people may be.

Fortunately, combination therapy is not harmful. We can try it with any patient who isn't feeling up to par with T4 therapy. I usually give combination therapy a six-month trial before assessing its value for a particular patient.

What Does the Literature Show?

Current medical literature on this topic is sparse and inconclusive. A one-year study in the 1970s treated patients for six months with combination therapy, then six months with T4 and a sugar pill (placebo) instead of T3. The patients did not know when they were on combination therapy and when they were on T4. Their TSH was maintained at about the same level in both six-month periods. At the end of the study, patients had to answer only one question: during which six-month period did you feel better? Most patients had no preference; among those who did, more people preferred T4 treatment to combination therapy.

The best-known study was published in *The New England Journal of Medicine* in 1999. It has been widely quoted by supporters of combination therapy. The research was conducted in Lithuania on 35 hypothyroid patients who had either thyroid cancer or Hashimoto's thyroiditis. The trial subjects were treated with T4 for five weeks and combination therapy for five weeks.

This was a randomized, double-blind trial, meaning that neither the patients nor the participating physicians knew which patients were taking T4 and which were on combination therapy in any given five-week interval. This is a generally preferred method of design for a clinical trial because it is thought to give the most unbiased results.

At the end of each period, patients underwent comprehensive thyroid tests and psychological assessment. The authors of the study concluded that:

- Combination therapy slightly improved patients' moods, ability to remember, and attention span.

- Most patients preferred combination therapy.

- All the laboratory tests, regardless of the therapy, were within the normal range.

The more recent study, published in 2005, attempted to replicate the results of the Lithuanian trials. Thirty patients underwent T4 and T4/T3 therapy for six weeks. However, the authors did not find any benefits from combination therapy. Both studies were small in the number of patients and were short in duration, so neither of them can be used as a definitive answer to the question of combination therapy. This shows how hard it is to find out what the best treatment is. Larger and better designed studies will be needed to answer this question.

In the largest study to date done in 1971, 141 patients were examined for 15 weeks in a similar fashion. Most preferred combination therapy to T4 treatment, but no significant differences were detected through objective measurements. This study included patients with TSH levels between 0.11 and 4.0, which means some of the patients were not adequately treated prior to the study.

There are several other published studies, but it would be redundant to describe all of them. The results were similar and remain controversial.

What Do I Think About Combination Therapy?

In my opinion, none of these studies were appropriately designed to answer the question about the benefits of combination therapy. More important, the patients studied were not properly selected.

I believe such a study should focus only on patients who are not feeling well on T4 therapy. Patients who are perfectly happy with their current therapy are highly unlikely to feel happier with a new treatment. Also, patients with thyroid cancer should not be included in such a study because they are treated with higher doses of T4 than are patients with garden-variety hypothyroidism.

Furthermore, patients should be kept on each therapy for at least six months for the effects to be accurately assessed. Five weeks, as in the Lithuanian study, is not enough time. The reason for this is that the studies themselves have an initial positive impact on patients: they tend to feel optimistic about the study's outcome, they are motivated to take their medication, and so forth. Most of these effects dissipate in a couple of months. After six months, only the pure effects of the therapy remain and can be accurately measured.

Until we have results from such a study, I will continue to prescribe combination therapy—on a six-month trial basis—for patients who don't feel up to speed when treated with T4 alone and whose TSH is below 2.0 milliunits per milliliter. Thus far, only a small number of my patients experienced improvement in their symptoms and wanted to continue combination therapy.

Controversy #3: Treating Mental Disorders with Thyroid Hormones

Remember Christopher from chapter 2? His family believed he had dementia, and he had been diagnosed with Alzheimer's disease, when in fact he suffered from profound hypothyroidism. People have been diagnosed and hospitalized for months for psychosis and other mental illnesses when they simply had under- or overactive thyroids.

The symptoms of hyperthyroidism and hypothyroidism overlap with those of many mental illnesses. Hyperthyroid patients are anxious, may exhibit sudden mood shifts, and can be extremely irritable and hyperactive. They may be acutely sensitive to noise and experience bouts of depression, insomnia, and loss of appetite. In extreme cases, they appear schizophrenic and out of touch with reality. They can become delirious and even hallucinate—all symptoms of mental illness.

Similarly, hypothyroidism can lead to a slowing of mental processes, short-term memory loss, depression with paranoid features, and progressive loss of interest and initiative in day-to-day life. Eventually, if not controlled, an underactive thyroid can cause a dementia-like state and permanent brain damage.

These are extreme situations, but I have seen at least two hyperthyroid patients who were unable to manage their lives before treatment. Both exhibited symptoms reminiscent of schizophrenia, and both recovered their mental abilities once their hyperthyroidism was controlled.

In my experience, psychiatrists are usually able to distinguish between patients who suffer from thyroid disease and those with mental illness. Nonetheless, I believe that patients with mental illnesses should always be tested for thyroid dysfunction.

Are Mental Illness and Thyroid Disease Linked?

Studies have examined the potential relationship between thyroid disease and mental illness. But it is still too early to prescribe definitive treatment based on the results of this research.

Women who have positive thyroid antibodies in early pregnancy are prone to postpartum depression. There appears to be a link between the two conditions. However, women's postpartum depression seems independent of their thyroid function. Blood tests frequently show that their free T4, free T3, and TSH levels are normal.

In one study of postpartum depression, 446 women were given 100 micrograms of T4 for six months after delivery. The women were checked for symptoms of depression every four weeks. Unfortunately, the researchers found no evidence to suggest that T4 had any effect on postpartum depression.

Treating Depression with Thyroid Hormones

Still, some psychiatrists treat depression and other mental illnesses with thyroid hormone—even when the patients' thyroids are healthy—in conjunction with antidepressants and other traditional psychiatric medications.

One reason for this is that some depressed patients do not respond to traditional treatment. This has led psychiatrists to experiment with supplemental therapies to augment the effects of antidepressants. One strategy is to add a second antidepressant. Other treatments include prescribing lithium, a medication used to treat more serious psychiatric diseases (psychoses and bipolar depression), stimulants, and so forth.

Since a shortage or overabundance of thyroid hormones affects mood, some psychiatrists prescribe T3 and T4 in cases of hard-to-treat depression; 25 to 30 percent of hard-to-treat depressed patients have shown improvement when T3 was administered in conjunction with antidepressants.

In some studies, depressed patients were given enough T3 and T4 supplements, in addition to antidepressants, to cause mild hyperthyroidism. Mood improvement was found in nearly 30 percent of patients. However, these studies were brief in duration, typically four weeks. It isn't certain that the beneficial effects would persist over the long term.

One study compared the side effects of mild hyperthyroidism induced by T4 therapy in healthy subjects and in patients suffering from depression. The authors of the study concluded that these side effects were less pronounced in the depressed patients. This suggests that mild hyperthyroidism may be better tolerated during depression than when a person is healthy. One could then hypothesize that keeping a depressed person hyperthyroid with medication may not be as harmful as doing so with someone who is not depressed. However, since long-term hyperthyroidism puts the heart and bones at risk, such a therapy should be administered only under the supervision of both a psychiatrist and an endocrinologist.

Despite these successes, we are still mostly in the dark about the role of thyroid hormones in the treatment of depression. We do not understand why thyroid hormone therapy helps some patients but not others. One possibility is that these patients actually have very mild thyroid dysfunction, which contributes to their depression. In these cases, thyroid hormone treatment actually corrects the underlying thyroid problem. On the other hand, sometimes a patient's depression is alleviated with such a small dose of thyroid hormones that it is difficult to believe that thyroid dysfunction could be so easily corrected.

We must admit that we do not always know how or why thyroid hormone treatment helps with depression.

Controversy #4: Body Temperature and "Wilson's Syndrome"

One of the symptoms of profound hypothyroidism is dramatic hypothermia (decreased body temperature). Some physicians have assumed that even a moderately low body temperature is a sign of hypothyroidism; I disagree.

A Florida physician named E. Denis Wilson built a treatment system around this belief. He claimed that a cluster of symptoms that include fatigue, hair loss, weight gain, diminished libido, poor memory, headaches, and moderately low body temperature, even when accompanied by normal hormone levels, constitute a type of thyroid dysfunction that he dubbed "Wilson's syndrome" or "Wilson's temperature syndrome."

He claimed that this breed of hypothyroidism is diagnosed by the appearance of a cluster of symptoms and an oral temperature reading of less than 98.6 degrees Fahrenheit. Obviously, Wilson's syndrome cannot be diagnosed by using standard thyroid tests since the syndrome is accompanied by normal hormone levels.

According to Wilson, the disorder must be treated by the "Wilson T3 regimen"—that is, by administering high daily doses of T3. This can be a dangerous treatment when given to patients who have normal hormone levels; it may induce hyperthyroidism. In 1991, one of Dr. Wilson's patients, a 50-year-old woman who was taking massive doses of T3, died from a rapid heartbeat (likely caused by his therapy).

The case was settled out of court for $250,000. In 1992, the Florida Board of Medicine fined Dr. Wilson, suspended his license for six months, and ordered him to undergo psychological testing. He has not resumed the practice of medicine. But his ideas are still promoted by the Wilson's Syndrome Foundation and its website.

Several practitioners of alternative medicine still claim to be able to treat Wilson's syndrome with T3. Some patients take more than 200 micrograms of T3 per day. (Remember that the normal daily dose is 25 to 50 micrograms.) Of course, these treatments require a hefty payment.

I have been asked by patients to prescribe T3 for treatment of Wilson's syndrome, but have declined to do so. I agree with the conclusions of the American Thyroid Association regarding Wilson's syndrome:

"The proposed basis of Wilson's syndrome is not consistent with well-known and accepted facts about thyroid hormone production, metabolism, and action.

"The diagnostic criteria for Wilson's syndrome are nonspecific and imprecise.

"There is no scientific evidence that T3 therapy is better than a placebo for management of these nonspecific symptoms in individuals with normal thyroid hormone levels.

"T3 therapy, as prescribed by promoters of Wilson's syndrome, results in wide fluctuations in T3 concentrations in blood and body tissues. This produces symptoms and cardiovascular complications in some patients, and is potentially dangerous."

Controversy #5: Goitrogens: Thyroid-Suppressing Foods

Doctors have known for a long time that some foods can induce thyroid enlargement if they are consumed in large quantities and for an extended period. These foods make it difficult for the thyroid to absorb iodine from the blood, causing a condition similar to iodine deficiency. An iodine shortage prevents the thyroid from manufacturing normal levels of thyroid hormones. The pituitary senses the shortfall and responds by increasing TSH levels. This stimulates the thyroid gland to grow and may cause a goiter.

Iodine-blocking foods are called goitrogens because they have the ability to induce goiters. There are two categories of goitrogen foods: foods made from soybeans and cruciferous vegetables like cauliflower and broccoli. Millet, peaches, and strawberries—although not in either of the above-mentioned categories—also contain goitrogens.

What Foods Are Considered Goitrogens?

Soybean-Related Foods. Soy foods contain isoflavones (part of compounds called flavonoids), which reduce thyroid hormone production. They do this by blocking the enzyme thyroid peroxidase from catalyzing oxidation of iodine atoms, which prevents them from attaching to thyroglobulin proteins to make T4 and T3. This is one of the few areas in which flavonoid intake has an adverse effect. Most research shows the beneficial properties of flavonoids; these naturally occurring phytonutrients have repeatedly been shown to support hearty health.

Soy foods with isoflavones include:

- Tofu
- Tempeh

- Miso (fermented soybean paste made into a traditional Japanese soup)
- Soy milk
- Soy flour
- Soy bread
- Soybean oil
- Soy nuts
- Soy cookies
- Soy sauce
- Tamari

Cruciferous Vegetables. Cruciferous vegetables contain isothiocyanates, which have been linked to decreased thyroid hormone production. Like isoflavones, isothiocyanates appear to block iodine uptake by the thyroid and disrupt messages telegraphed across the membranes of thyroid cells.

Cruciferous vegetables include:

- Broccoli
- Cauliflower
- Brussels sprouts
- Cabbage
- Mustard
- Kale
- Turnips
- Rapeseed (canola oil)
- Kohlrabi
- African cassava
- Rutabaga

Other Foods. Other foods that contain goitrogens include:

- Peaches
- Peanuts
- Millet
- Spinach
- Strawberries
- Radishes

Are These Foods Really Dangerous?

A great deal has been written about the effects of goitrogen-laden foods on human health. Some literature suggests that consuming these foods is a major health risk. However, in the absence of thyroid disease, there is no convincing data that goitrogen-containing foods have a negative impact on health. In fact, the opposite appears to be true: Soy products and cruciferous vegetables have unique nutritional values. Studies have repeatedly shown that eating these foods decreases the risk of contracting a wide array of diseases.

But there is controversy in the medical world about whether patients with thyroid disease, especially patients with hypothyroidism, should eat foods containing goitrogens. To date, no well-designed scientific study has examined this issue.

Health care providers' opinions differ widely as to whether a person who has a thyroid hormone deficiency should limit intake of goitrogenic foods. Most recommend avoidance of overconsumption or excessive intake. Usually, the goal is to limit intake but not to eliminate goitrogenic foods completely from the diet.

Personally, I do not recommend limiting goitrogens in the diets of patients being treated for hypothyroidism for two reasons:

1. Their metabolisms no longer rely on their thyroid glands since we are supplying their hormone needs with synthesized

T4. (Blocking hormone production in an already inactive thyroid has virtually no effect.) Their TSH has been normalized, and they are not at risk for developing goiter.

2. I consider it prudent to include these foods in a meal plan because of their strong nutritional value and their outstanding track record in preventing many other health problems.

However, I do recommend limiting goitrogen intake for patients who already have enlarged thyroids, though I still would not advise eliminating them from the diet altogether.

The truth is, in areas where iodine intake is sufficient, you must consume large quantities of goitrogens to affect thyroid hormone production. Since iodine intake is adequate in the common American diet, goitrogens are not overly harmful.

In addition, both isoflavones (found in soy foods) and isothiocyanates (contained in cruciferous vegetables) are heat-sensitive. Cooking will destroy about one-third of these substances.

The situation is far different in areas like central Africa (far from the sea), where iodine intake is low and goitrogen intake is high. The goitrogen African cassava, for example, is widely consumed in central Africa. Since diets are not rich in iodine in this part of the world, and goitrogens are widely consumed, thyroid hormone production can be limited. Under these circumstances, goitrogens will enlarge the thyroid gland. It is no wonder that goiters are still a major concern in this area.

Controversy #6: Thyroid and Fibromyalgia

I am sure most readers have heard of fibromyalgia, a chronic condition characterized by fatigue; widespread pain in the muscles, ligaments, and tendons; and multiple tender points—places on the body where even slight pressure causes pain. In the past, this condition was known by names such as fibrositis, chronic muscle pain syndrome, psychogenic rheumatism, and tension myalgia. It is believed that between three million and eight million Americans suffer from fibromyalgia; 80 to 90 percent of them are women.

Signs and symptoms of fibromyalgia fluctuate, depending on the weather, stress, physical activity, and even the time of day. The most common are:

- Pain occurring in localized areas of the body when pressure is applied: in the back of the head, the upper back and neck, the upper chest, elbows, hips, and knees. This pain generally persists for months and is often accompanied by stiffness.

- Waking up tired even after plenty of sleep. Some studies suggest that people with fibromyalgia miss the deep, restorative stage of sleep.

- Nighttime muscle spasms (charley horses) in the legs. Restless legs syndrome may also be associated with fibromyalgia.

- Constipation, diarrhea, abdominal pain, and bloating, which are associated with irritable bowel syndrome.

- Many fibromyalgia patients have headaches and facial pain, which is linked to tenderness or stiffness in their neck and shoulders. Dysfunction of the jaw joints and surrounding muscles is another common feature.

- Sensitivity to odors, noises, and bright lights

Other signs and symptoms include:

- Depression
- Numbness or tingling sensations in the hands and feet (paresthesias)
- Difficulty concentrating

- Chest pain
- Irritable bladder
- Dry eyes, skin, and mouth
- Painful menstrual periods
- Dizziness
- Anxiety

Many of these symptoms are also features of hypothyroidism. This has led some practitioners to assert that all fibromyalgia patients suffer from hypothyroidism, even those with normal thyroid functions. They propose treating fibromyalgia patients with thyroid hormones. I do not agree.

Over the years, I have encountered a few patients diagnosed with fibromyalgia. But when they were diagnosed and treated for hypothyroidism, their fibromyalgia symptoms disappeared. It is clear to me that these patients were originally misdiagnosed; their hypothyroid symptoms were confused with those of fibromyalgia.

My position is that every patient who has the symptoms of fibromyalgia should be tested for thyroid dysfunction. If even a minor thyroid abnormality is detected, it should be corrected before a diagnosis of fibromyalgia is considered.

Controversy #7: Unproven Thyroid Supplements

The Internet abounds with websites that promote a wide variety of health supplements, including preparations purported to relieve thyroid disorders. But none of these has been proved effective. I attempt to keep up with online therapies, but it is difficult to know them all. Here are my thoughts on some of the most common offerings.

Thyroid Helper

Thyroid Helper is a preparation that supposedly provides supplementation of selenium, manganese, tyrosine, ashwagandha (an Ayurvedic herb), and gugulipids. (Ayurveda is an ancient system of medicine practiced extensively in Sri Lanka and India. Gugulipids are preparations made from the resin of the mukul myrrh tree, which grows in India. The tree's resin is called gum guggul or guggulu.)

According to the website *www.wellnessresources.com*, Thyroid Helper is designed to boost metabolism by resolving issues that block T4 to T3 conversion. According to this site, anyone who has difficulty losing weight is most likely experiencing a sluggish thyroid.

Also, according to the manufacturer, selenium enables the body to convert T4 to T3, and manganese will help with weight gain on the hips and thighs. The makers state, correctly, that tyrosine is needed to make thyroid hormones; but in addition, they credit the amino acid with the ability to nourish the sympathetic nervous system. They contend that the ashwagandha herb has been shown to reduce liver stress and increase levels of T3, and they claim that gugulipids lower LDL cholesterol (bad cholesterol) by 25 percent and increase HDL cholesterol (good cholesterol) by 35 percent.

This product is available at a discounted price of $18 for 90 capsules. The recommended dose is 1 to 2 capsules with each meal (3 to 6 capsules a day).

Selenium

Selenium is an essential trace mineral. It is found naturally in seafood, liver, lean red meat, and grains grown in selenium-rich soil. Selenium helps prevent cell damage caused by oxidants, highly reactive molecules containing oxygen, which damage normal molecules.

Several studies suggest that a deficiency of selenium can lead to health problems, including thyroid disease. It appears that severe selenium deficiency increases the death rate of thyroid cells, which are then replaced by connective tissue (scar).

But these are merely observational studies. They measure the prevalence of selenium deficiency that is associated with thyroid disorders in a given population. Observational studies cannot prove that one feature triggers another and therefore cannot show that selenium causes thyroid dysfunction. However, the results of these preliminary studies indicate the need for further research in this area.

In the United States, selenium deficiency is extremely rare. Selenium toxicity, though also rare, is more common. Selenium toxicity was first described in the 13th century in China when cattle and horses experienced adverse reactions after eating plants containing large amounts of selenium. The animals suffered from hair loss—especially the mane and tails of the horses and the tail switches of the cattle—as well as hoof deformities and sores.

Humans with selenium toxicity (selenosis) also experience hair loss as well as brittle nails. Other symptoms include fatigue, irritability, skin rash, sour-milk or garlic-like breath odor, nausea, and vomiting.

A well-known case of selenium toxicity occurred in 1984. A 57-year-old woman started shedding her hair less than two weeks after beginning selenium supplements. In two months, she was nearly bald! She also developed whitish streaking on one fingernail, tenderness and swelling of her fingertips, and pus discharge under the nails. Eventually, she lost a fingernail. In addition, she experienced nausea, vomiting, sour-milk breath odor, and fatigue.

Other people who took the pills suffered similar symptoms. Hair loss and fingernail aberrations (horizontal streaking, blackening of the nails, and nail loss) were the most common. Finally, it was discovered that the selenium tablets contained about 27 milligrams of selenium—182 times more than advertised! The product was recalled by the distributor.

Daily consumption of 3.20 to 6.69 milligrams of selenium by individuals in China also produced loss of hair and nails, skin rash, garlic breath, fatigue, irritability, and increased muscle reflexes.

The recommended dietary allowance (RDA) of selenium is 55 micrograms per day for adults, 60 micrograms for pregnant women, and 70 micrograms for lactating women.

A safe adult dosage appears to be not more than 900 micrograms per day. Prolonged intake of more than 1,000 micrograms (or 1 milligram) daily may cause adverse reactions.

Coconut Oil

Coconut oil has been marketed as a thyroid function booster. I could not determine the exact mechanism for its presumed effect, but in researching coconut oil literature, I found many published opinions of self-proclaimed experts as well as four bona fide studies that examined the effects of coconut oil on the body.

In these tests, coconut oil was used as a source of medium-chain fatty acids. Medium-chain fatty acids metabolize faster than the long-chain fatty acids found in most vegetable and fish oils and have been studied in other contexts for their possible role in preventing and curing obesity. The coconut-oil studies showed that subjects had somewhat greater energy expenditure when most of the fat in their diets derived from medium-chain fatty acids rather than long-chain fatty acids.

This finding suggests that consuming more medium-chain fatty acids, like those found in coconut oil, can boost weight-loss efforts. However, the only study that followed participants for more than a day or two found that these effects are present seven days after taking coconut oil but disappear by day 14.

I could not find any published data on the specific effects of coconut oil on thyroid function and could not glean any supporting evidence for the claim that coconut oil is beneficial for patients suffering from thyroid disorder. Of course, there are plenty of testimonials from happy customers that could not be verified.

You can purchase a quart of coconut oil online for $30 to $60.

Estro Thin

Estro Thin is sold primarily for postmenopausal symptoms. But it has also been marketed on the Web as a supplement for patients with thyroid diseases.

This concoction contains many herbal extracts that allegedly increase energy levels, lower blood sugar, improve concentration, strengthen the immune system, decrease appetite, and perform other happy functions. But curiously, there is no mention of any effect on the thyroid. One wonders why it is marketed as a thyroid product.

The official Estro Thin website (*www.estrothin.com*) states,

> *Weight control, how much energy people have, how well they get up in the morning, how well they sleep, and how much stamina they have for the day is [sic] directly related to their levels of thyroid hormone. When your thyroid level is too low, you don't have the energy to cope adequately with anything, much less the additional stress and emotional liability associated with the menopausal years.*
>
> *Menopause is not an illness, but it can begin to feel that way if your thyroid is low or borderline at the time of your change . . . supplementation of Estro Thin can help"* (Estro Thin, *"Thyroid Function,"* www.estrothin.com/thyroid.php, *accessed October 5, 2008).*

The website claims the product will:

• Help support thyroid function

• Help increase metabolic rate and the number of calories burned

- Help control appetite
- Help relieve other menopause and thyroid symptoms

If you buy two bottles at $99.90, the third is free. A single bottle sells for $49.95.

Metabolic Thyro

According to the website that sells it (*www.doctorsresearch.com*), this preparation contains alfalfa, bovine (cow) adrenal concentrate, bovine liver concentrate, bovine pituitary concentrate, bovine thyroid concentrate, burdock root, guar gum seed, kelp thallus, L-tyrosine, plant polysaccharides, and skullcap herb. It supposedly provides a nutritional supplement for the thyroid.

I was unable to determine the recommended daily dose, but before using this preparation, please reread the section in chapter 4 of this book about factitious hyperthyroidism. You may recall that people in three states became hyperthyroid after accidentally eating bovine thyroid tissue that was ground up in their hamburgers. Ninety pills cost $19.98.

Warning: Bovine products may carry the risk of Creutzfeldt-Jakob disease, a human form of mad cow disease.

Thyroid Assist

According to the website that sells it (*www.nativeremedies.com*), Thyroid Assist is a supplement that remedies iodine deficiency (a problem rarely found in the United States). It contains sea kelp as a source of iodine and wild oat plant, which supposedly supports nerve function, increases libido, helps combat hypothyroidism, and lowers cholesterol. It also contains an herb from the mint family, used in Ayurvedic medicine, as a remedy for high blood pressure and hypothyroidism.

A 50-milliliter bottle costs $36.95.

Bugleweed-Motherwort Compound

According to the website that sells it (*www.herb-pharm.com*), this preparation helps alleviate overactive thyroid conditions. The manufacturer includes a disclaimer, stating that it cannot recommend the preparation in place of medical treatments and that the compound may not be compatible with traditional drugs used to treat hyperthyroidism—which I find a rather contradictory position.

According to the manufacturer, this product is safe for long-term treatment. A four-ounce bottle lasts about one month. It is taken with 30 to 50 drops in water, three to five times daily.

The product contains a blend of the liquid extracts of:

- Bugleweed flowering herb
- Motherwort flowering tops
- Cactus stem
- Lemon balm leaf and flower

Herbs are either certified organically grown or wild-crafted. The base is partially pharmaceutical-grade grain alcohol.

A four-ounce bottle runs $41.50.

And There Are Many More . . .

These are only a handful of the preparations that can be purchased online. The others, for the most part, contain the same ingredients as the above preparations. It would be redundant to list all of them.

In my opinion, there is no convincing data that any of these preparations are appropriate treatment for thyroid disorders. I believe that serious thyroid conditions require standard treatment therapies.

Would I advise against the use of these preparations? If patients feel better while taking any of them, I would not object to their continued usage. On the other hand, I am not certain that all of these products are safe. Some of them are decidedly unsafe. Also, they may be safe taken alone but unsafe taken with traditional thyroid medications. We just don't know.

I make sure my patients understand that I do not endorse any of these preparations.

Conclusion

Thyroid disorders are common, but we have good tools to diagnose and treat them. I hope this book provided you with enough information to recognize situations in which your thyroid should be checked.

Sometimes the thyroid throws us a curve ball and requires more complex diagnostic and therapeutic measures than are usually sufficient. Very rarely will I find a patient who defies my understanding of thyroid physiology, but it has happened. I once had a patient who took 12 micrograms of T4 and felt poorly with a higher or lower dose. I did not understand how this particular dose was helping her, but I trusted that it helped her. Or consider my patient who seemingly could not absorb any of the thyroid hormone in any form I gave her. She is now treated with injections of T4 into the muscle twice a week.

An open mind helps me learn from my patients and helps me help my patients.

Inflexible Treatment Programs

We are inundated with "expert" opinions regarding thyroid treatment from newspapers, the Internet, books, and self-help magazines. Although these opinions often conflict, each "expert" seems convinced that his or her advice is correct. Many claim that their thyroid treatment is the best therapy for all patients.

I believe most of these individuals are honest and want to be helpful. However, the human body is inordinately complex, and people differ in their responses to illness and to treatment. Most differences in the broad spectrum of possible responses are unknown to both alternative healers and modern science. It is irresponsible to push a single viewpoint and approach as the solution to all thyroid problems. Frequently, inflexible medical opinions are anchored in limited personal experience or a handful of cases.

I have heard many accounts of doctors who prescribe one mode of therapy and regard all others as inferior or suspect. I am wary of such practitioners, who insist upon a single therapy and require their patients to adhere to it or find another physician. In such cases, I would strongly recommend finding another doctor.

Some patients plead with me not to send a letter to their regular doctors because they have visited me without their knowledge, and the doctors apparently would not accept a diagnosis or treatment plan that differed from their own. If you are uncomfortable telling your doctor about a visit to a specialist, he or she should not be your doctor. There must be a relationship of mutual trust and openness between patients and their doctors, and a good physician knows when it is time to send his or her patient to a specialist.

My approach is to begin by admitting to patients that my assessments may be wrong. The doctrine of medical infallibility is a myth, left over from earlier eras. I frequently promise my patients that if I fail to help them, it will not be for lack of trying—meaning that I am willing to administer a wide variety of therapies. The final determinant of which therapy works best is the patient's response to treatment.

I avoid any therapy that I consider risky for a particular patient (such as maintaining the TSH below a detectable level). But within the limits of safety, I am open to all forms of therapy. Ultimately, I allow patients to decide which treatment best suits their needs.

My advice to all patients is to find a doctor who will listen and is open to a wide array of opinions. Such doctors exist, and it is worth any effort to track them down. After all, you would look for another auto mechanic if you were not satisfied with the one you had, wouldn't you?

Index

About the Author

Mario Skugor, MD, is a staff endocrinologist at Cleveland Clinic. He is an Associate Professor of Medicine and director of Endocrinology Block at Cleveland Clinic Lerner College of Medicine of CWRU. He is also a associate Director of Endocrinology, Diabetes and Metabolism Fellowship at Cleveland Clinic. He got his Medical Degree at University of Zagreb in Croatia. He had his postgraduate training at University Hospitals of Zagreb in Croatia, St Luke's Medical Center in Cleveland and at Cleveland Clinic. His main areas of interest are thyroid disorders, diabetes mellitus, obesity and disorders of calcium metabolism.